# Towards Effective Disease Control in Ghana

## RESEARCH AND POLICY IMPLICATIONS

Volume 2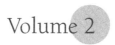

### NOGUCHI READER

Editors

**Kwadwo A. Koram**

**Collins K. Ahorlu**

**Michael D. Wilson**

**Dorothy Yeboah-Manu**

**Kwabena M. Bosompem**

**UNIVERSITY OF GHANA READERS**

CLINICAL SCIENCES SERIES NO 5 ( Volume 2)

First published in Ghana 2014 for THE UNIVERSITY OF GHANA
by **Sub-Saharan Publishers**
P.O.Box 358
Legon-Accra
Ghana
Email: saharanp@africaonline.com.gh

© University of Ghana, 2014,
P.O.Box LG 25
Legon- Accra
Ghana
Tel: +233-302-500381
website:http://www.ug.edu.gh

ISBN: 978-9988-647-62-9

# Contents

# List of Tables

# List of Figures

# Foreword

The University of Ghana is celebrating this year the sixty-fifth anniversary of its founding. In all those years, lecturers and researchers of the university have contributed in quite significant ways to the development of thought and to the analysis of critical issues for different aspects of Ghanaian and African society. The celebration of the anniversary provides an appropriate opportunity for reflection on the contributions that Legon academics have made to the intellectual development of Ghana and Africa. That is what this Readers Project is about.

In the early years of the University, all the material that was used to teach students came largely from the United Kingdom and other parts of Europe. Most of the thinking in all disciplines was largely Eurocentric. The material that was used to teach students was mainly European, as indeed were many of the people teaching the students. The norms and standards against which students were assessed were influenced largely by European values. The discussions that took place in seminar and lecture rooms were driven largely by what Africa could learn from Europe.

The 1960s saw a major 'revision' in African intellectual development as young African academics began to question received ideas against a backdrop of changing global attitudes in the wake of political independence. Much serious writing was done by African academics as their contribution to the search for new ways of organizing their societies. African intellectuals contributed to global debates in their own right and sometimes developed their own material for engaging with their students and the wider society.

Since the late 1970s universities in the region and their academics have struggled to make their voices heard in national and global debates. In a context of economic stagnation and political disarray, many of the ideas for managing African economies and societies have come from outside. These ideas have often come with significant financial backing channeled through international organizations and governments. During the period, African governments saw themselves as having no reason to expect or ask for any intellectual contribution from their own academics. This was very much the case in Ghana, as indeed in most African countries.

The story is beginning to change in many African universities. The Readers Project at the University of Ghana, Legon is an attempt to document the different ideas that have influenced various disciplines over many years. Through collections of short essays, they are also an illustration of the debates that have emerged over the years. They show the work of Legon academics and their collaborators in various disciplines as they have sought to introduce their students to new ideas. Our expectation is that this will mark a new beginning of solid engagement between Legon and other academics as they document their thoughts and contributions to the continuing search for new ideas to shape our world.

We gratefully acknowledge a generous grant from the Carnegie Corporation of New York that has made the publication of this series of Readers possible.

**Ernest Aryeetey**
*Vice-Chancellor, University of Ghana.*
Legon, August 2013

# List of Contributors (Volumes 1 and 2)

**Anthony Ablordey** (PhD) is a Senior Research Fellow in the Bacteriology Department of the Noguchi Memorial Institute for Medical Research, University of Ghana. Dr. Ablordey was part of an international team of Scientists that successfully cultivated *Mycobacterium ulcerans* from the environment for the first time. *Research interests*: Molecular epidemiology and control of Buruli ulcer disease.

**Benjamin Abuaku** (PhD) is a Research Fellow in the Department of Epidemiology, Noguchi Memorial Institute for Medical Research. *Research interests*: malaria epidemiology, tuberculosis treatment outcomes, obesity and impact of floods on health.

**Stephanie Kabukwor Adjovu** (MPhil) is a Research Assistant at the Parasitology Department of the Noguchi Memorial Institute for Medical Research. *Research interests*: helminthiasis, malaria, emerging molecular and diagnostic tools for parasitic infections, health promotion, and evaluation and monitoring, and policy change biomedical research.

**Innocent Afeke** (MPhil) is a Microbiologist/Medical Laboratory Technologist in the Animal Experimentation Department of Noguchi Memorial Institute for Medical Research. *Research interests*: the reservoir and mode of transmission of *Mycobacterium ulcerans*, etiologic agent of Buruli ulcer.

**Collins S.K. Ahorlu** (PhD) is a Senior Research Fellow and head of the Epidemiology Department of the Noguchi Memorial Institute for Medical Research. *Research interests*: socio-cultural and epidemiology of malaria, TB, filariasis and Buruli ulcer, adolescent sexual and reproductive health, implementation research and leadership.

**Nana Ama Amissah** (MPhil) is a Senior Research Assistant in the Bacteriology Department of the Noguchi Memorial Institute for Medical Research, University of Ghana. *Research interests*: investigating the role of free living amebae as host of Mycrobacterium ulcerans; Buruli ulcer control activities.

**Linda Eva Amoah** (PhD) is a Research Fellow in the Immunology Department.

*Research interests*: understanding how transmission-blocking immunity against malaria is developed amongst genetically diverse individuals and the biology of *Plasmodium falciparum* gametocytes designing and producing malaria antigens for serology and vaccinology.

**William Kwabena Ampofo** (PhD) is an Associate Professor and head of the Virology Department. He is currently the Head of the National Influenza Centre.

*Research interests:* in molecular and serological investigations and prevention of viral infections, anti-viral chemotherapy and epidemiological investigations of viral disease burden.

**Nii-Ayi Ankrah** (PhD) is an Associate Professor, Clinical Chemistry/Toxicology in the Department of Clinical Pathology, Noguchi Memorial Institute for Medical Research, University of Ghana, Legon.

*Research interests:* environmental health, focusing on health effects of mycotoxins (aflatoxins), heavy metals (lead and mercury) and the antioxidant, glutathione.

**William Kofi Anyan** (PhD) is a Research Fellow at the Parasitology Department of Noguchi Memorial Institute for Medical Research.

*Research interests*: schistosomiasis control through understanding of transmission dynamics, the development of alternative drugs and identification of antigen candidates for vaccine developments.

**Maxwell A. Appawu** (PhD) is a Medical Entomologist/Parasitologist and a Senior Research Fellow in the Parasitology Department of the Noguchi Memorial Institute for Medical Research.

*Research interests:* the biology, epidemiology and control of vector-borne diseases with emphasis on transmission of malaria, dengue and yellow fever, leishmaniasis, filariasis, and the development of novel approaches for mosquito control.

**Regina Appiah-Opong** (PhD), Biochemist/Toxicologist, is a Research Fellow at the Clinical Pathology Department, Noguchi Memorial Institute for Medical Research.

*Research interests*: molecular toxicology, investing pharmacokinetic drug-drug, herb-drug and food-drug interactions at the level of cytochrome P450 enzymes and glutathione transferases, and drug development from plant sources.

**Daniel Kojo Arhinful** (PhD) is a Research Fellow of the Epidemiology Department. He was the Country Scientific Research Coordinator of the Immpact Project.

*Research interests*: access to medicines, social health insurance, social security and migrants, maternal and child health and chronic diseases in African populations.

**George Enyimah Armah** (PhD) is an Associate Professor at the Department of Electron Microscopy and Histopathology. He is also the Head of the West African Regional Rotavirus Reference Laboratory.

*Research interests*: enteric viruses, with particular interest in rotaviruses and noroviruses.

**Margaret Armar-Klemesu** (PhD) is an Associate Professor in the Department of Nutrition. She was Country Technical Partner Leader for Immpact.

*Research interests*: maternal and child health and nutrition, including programme design and evaluation, livelihoods and food security assessment and micronutrient interventions.

**Andy Asafu–Adjaye** (BSc) is a Senior Research Assistant in the Parasitology Department of the Noguchi Memorial Institute for Medical Research.

*Research interests*: medical entomology and modules for various neglected tropical diseases like malaria and lymphatic filariasis.

**Adwoa Asante-Poku** (MPhil) is a Principal Research Assistant with the Bacteriology Department. She is currently pursuing a PhD in microbiology at the Swiss Tropical and Public Health Institute, University of Basel.

*Research interests:* understanding the genetic diversity among members of the Mycobacterium tuberculosis complex circulating in Ghana; the genetic diversity and associated risk factors for TB such as co-morbidity with HIV and diabetes as well as drug resistance.

**Jonas R. K. Asigbee** was a Superintendent Technologist in the Parasitology Department of the Noguchi Memorial Institute for Medical Research. He served as a technical expert in several national and international training programmes.
*Research interests*: parasitic diseases.

**Irene Ayi** (PhD) is a Research Fellow and currently the Ag. Head of Parasitology Department, and Programme Manager of WACIPAC at the Noguchi Memorial Institute for Medical Research.
*Research interests*: transmission, prevention and control of neglected tropical parasitic disease and zoonotic diseases of public health importance.

**Langbong Bimi** (PhD) is a Senior Lecturer at the Department of Animal Biology and Conservation Science, University of Ghana.
*Research interests*: the epidemiology of tropical and parasitic diseases; the impact of water and sanitation on human health.

**Daniel Adjei Boakye** (PhD) is a Professor of parasitology at the Institute. He specializes in vector-borne diseases and allergic disorders.
*Researh interests*; challenges of control, diagnostics and climate change related to NTDs and malaria; the role of parasitic infections in allergic disorders.

**Daniel Boamah** (PhD) is a Research Officer at the Centre for Scientific Research into Plant Medicine (CSRPM), Mampong.
*Research interests*; immunology, bacteriology, parasitology, molecular biology, epidemiology, proteomics and bioinformatics of infectious diseases.

**J. H. Kofi Bonney** (PhD) is a Research Fellow in the Virology Department of the Noguchi Memorial Institute for Medical Research, University of Ghana.
*Research interests*; molecular and serological investigation of viral agents of emerging and dangerous pathogens; laboratory investigations; surveillance of viral hepatitis; respiratory tract infections of viral origin.

**Frank A. Bonsu** (MB. ChB, MPH, MSc) is the Director of the National TB Control Programme, Ghana Health Service and a part-time Lecturer at the School of Public Health, University of Ghana.

*Research interests*: infectious diseases, with a special focus on Tuberculosis.

**Kwabena Mante Bosompem** (PhD) is currently the Deputy Director at the NMIMR. Prof. Bosompem is the President of Community Directed Development Foundation (CDDF), and also President of the Ghana Red Cross Society (GRCS).

*Research interests*: development and integration of accurate diagnosis, vaccine research and advancing one's health; developing social systems, strategic partnerships and strengthening local governance for safety nets, livelihoods and participation.

**Samuel Kweku Dadzie** (PhD) is a Research Fellow in the Parasitology Department of the Noguchi Memorial Institute for Medical Research.

*Research interests*: vector biology with emphasis on the application of modern methods to address the biology of vector-borne diseases, vector population genetics, and the molecular genetics of insecticide resistance.

**Emmanuel Kakra Dickson** (BSc) is the Senior Technologist with the Department of Immunology.

*Research interests*: malaria diagnosis and epidemiology.

**Alfred Dodoo** (Msc) is a Chief Research Assistant in the Department of Electron Microscopy and Histopathology of the Noguchi Memorial Institute for Medical Research.

*Research interests*: experimental pathology of infectious diseases, ultrastructural and histological changes of cells/tissues interacting with pathogenic mycobacteria or parasitic protozoan.

**Daniel Dodoo**, (PhD) is an Associate Professor, Department of Immunology.

*Research interests*: malaria vaccine development and identification of antigens involved in protection against malaria, elucidation of immune mechanisms involved in acquisition of immunity and establishment of assays that are important for pre-clinical and clinical assessment of immunity.

**Nancy Odurowah Duah** (PhD) is a Research Fellow in the Epidemiology Department.

*Research interests*: antimalarial drug resistance monitoring, particularly in the molecular investigation of genetic markers associated with drug resistance in *Plasmodium falciparum*.

**Anita Ghansah** (PhD) is a Research Fellow in the Parasitology Department of the Noguchi Memorial Institute for Medical *Research*.

*Research interests*: genetic diversity and its influence on the epidemiology and pathogenicity of malaria; population genetics strategies to identify genetic loci that contribute to drug resistance in *P. falciparum* and the development of genomic tools to characterize *P. falciparum* diversity.

**Linnie Golightly** (MD) is an Associate Professor of Clinical Medicine, Microbiology and Immunology, Weill Medical College of Cornell University, New York, USA. She forged a cross-disciplinary collaboration between experts in microvascular repair at Cornell and malaria pathogenesis at the NMIMR at Legon to test the hypothesis that endothelial progenitor cells might be important in the pathogenesis of cerebral malaria.

**Ben Gyan** (PhD) is an Associate Professor Senior Research Fellow in the Immunology Department of the Noguchi Memorial Institute for Medical Research.

*Research interests*: identification of novel biological markers and their mechanisms in the pathogenesis of malaria and other diseases, characterization of the effect of genetic polymorphisms in cytokines and haptoglobin, the role of haptoglobin phenotypes in the outcome of diabetes and hypertension, characterizing the immune correlates against malaria and malaria vaccine trials.

**Eric Koka** (MPhil) is a Principal Research Assistant in the Epidemiology Department and currently a PhD student at the School of Public Health, University of Ghana.

*Research interests*: include sociocultural aspects of HIV/AIDS including stigma and discrimination, Buruli ulcer and reproductive health.

**Kwadwo Ansah Koram** (MBChB; MPH&TM; PhD; FGCP) is Professor of Epidemiology and currently, the Director of the Noguchi Memorial Institute for Medical Research. He is a public health physician with an interest in the epidemiology and control of malaria. He has been a part-time lecturer in epidemiology at the School of Public Health.

*Research interests*: epidemiology of drug resistant *Plasmodium falciparum* infections, and clinical trials in malaria and breast cancer.

**Seth Kumordzi** (MPhil) is a Research Assistant in the Epidemiology Department.

*Research interests*: in social, cultural and economic aspects of infectious disease of public health interest in Ghana, and health systems.

**Kwadwo Asamoah Kusi** (PhD) is a Research/Postdoctoral Fellow in the Immunology Department of the Noguchi Memorial Institute for Medical Research.

*Research interests*: malaria immunology, pathogenesis and vaccine development; immunology and etiology of parasite/viral co-infections and various cancers.

**Eric Kyei-Bafour** (BSc) is a Research Assistant with the Immunology Department of the Noguchi Memorial Institute for Medical Research.

*Research interests*: in malaria diagnosis and epidemiology.

**Barbara Mallet** (BSc) was a Senior Research Assistant on the Initiative for Maternal Mortality Programme Assessment (IMMPACT) project at the Noguchi Memorial Institute for Medical Research, Legon.

**Alexander Nyarko** (PhD), Fellow of the Ghana Academy of Arts and Sciences, is currently the Acting Dean of the University of Ghana School of Pharmacy.

*Research interests*: drug/chemical-induced toxic injury, clinical biochemistry, pharmacology and toxicology of phytomedicines, including anti-cancer drug discovery research.

**Evangeline Obodai** (MPhil) is a research scientist in the Department of Virology. She is currently undertaking her PhD on RSV infection in children.

*Research interests*: molecular identification and characterization of entero and respiratory viruses.

**John Kofi Odoom** (PhD) is a Research Fellow in the Department of Virology.

*Research interests*: molecular epidemiology; characterisation of polioviruses circulating in Ghana and the African region; determination of the different serotypes of enteroviruses that are in circulation in patients, healthy children and the environment and serological investigations of viral disease.

**Isaac Darko Otchere** (MPhil) is a Principal Research Assistant working on a Wellcome Trust tuberculosis project at the Bacteriology Department of the Noguchi Memorial Institute for Medical Research.

*Research interests*: comparative genomics and genome diversity between *Mycobacterium tuberculosis sensu stricto and Mycobacterium africanum*.

**Michael Fokuo Ofori** (PhD) is a Senior Research Fellow in the Immunology Department of the Noguchi Memorial Institute for Medical Research. He is currently, the Acting Head of the Electron Microscopy/Histology Department.

*Research interests*: malaria immunology, specifically in understanding the development of natural immune response to malaria in children and pregnant women with special interest in variant surface antigens as possible vaccine candidates.

**Joseph Otchere** (MPhil) is a Chief Research Assistant with the Parasitology Department, Noguchi Memorial Institute for Medical Research.

*Research interests*: malaria and neglected tropical diseases, such as lymphatic filariasis, schistosomiasis and soil-transmitted helminthiasis, epidemiology and molecular mechanisms of anthelminthic treatment failure in Kintampo North Municipality.

**Mark Ofosuhene** (PhD) is a Research Fellow at the Department of Clinical Pathology, Noguchi Memorial Institute for Medical Research, University of Ghana, Legon.

*Research interests*: efficacy and toxicity evaluations of phytomedicines/natural products to manage diabetes mellitus, malaria and erectile dysfunction, and studies of biochemical changes that are associated with these conditions.

**Mubarak Osei-Kwasi** (PhD) is a retired Senior Research Fellow of the Virology department, Noguchi Memorial Institute for Medical Research, University of Ghana.

*Research interests*: HIV, polio, measles and yellow fever.

**Sellase Pi-Bansa** (BSc) is a Senior Research Assistant in the Parasitology Department of the Noguchi Memorial Institute for Medical Research.

*Research interests*: malaria transmission, vectors of the disease and their resistance to insecticides.

**Joseph Kwatei Quartey** (BSc) is a Senior Technician at the Parasitology Department of the Noguchi Memorial Institute for Medical Research.

*Research interests*: schistosomiasis, lymphatic filariasis, soil transmitted helminthes and malaria vectors control, mass drug treatment in school-aged children.

**Isaac Quaye** (PhD) is an Associate Professor in Biochemistry at University of Namibia.

*Research interests:* the role of the antioxidant haptoglobin in the pathogenesis of malaria, diabetes and other diseases.

**Lydia Quaye** (MSc) is a Chief Nursing Officer in the Department of Epidemiology, Noguchi Memorial Institute for Medical Research.

*Research interests*: malaria epidemiological studies including vaccine trials and antimalarial drug efficacy surveillance.

**Ato Kwamena Tetteh** (MPhil) is currently a Biomedical Laboratory Scientist at the Cape Coast Metropolitan Hospital.

*Research interests*: control of tropical diseases, especially, malaria, schistosomiasis and intestinal helminthiasis.

**Michael D. Wilson** (PhD) is a Professor of Parasitology in the Parasitology Department of the Noguchi Memorial Institute for Medical Research, University of Ghana. He was a former Director of the Noguchi Memorial Institute for Medical Research, University of Ghana.

*Research interests*: sustainable control of neglected tropical diseases.

**Dorothy Yeboah-Manu** (PhD) is an Associate Professor and Head of the Bacteriology Department, Noguchi Memorial Institute for Medical Research.

*Research interests*: host-pathogen interactions in *Mycobacterium tuberculosis and Mycobacterium ulcerans* infections (understanding genomic diversity and the contribution to host immune response and virulence; epidemiology and transmission dynamics; and improvement of diagnostics).

**Sawudatu Zakariah-Akoto** (MPhil) is a Chief Research Assistant at the Nutrition Department of the Noguchi Memorial Institute for Medical Research. She is currently undertaking doctoral studies on the use of instant fortified complementary foods and the safety of drinking water in Ghana.

*Research interests*: infant health and nutrition, maternal health, urban food/nutrition and livelihood security issues, urban agriculture and HIV/AIDS.

# Chapter 10
## Tuberculosis (TB): Local Solutions for a Global Public Health Problem

*Dorothy Yeboah-Manu, Adwoa Asante-Poku, Isaac Darko Otchere, Frank Bonsu and Collins K. Ahorlu*

## Introduction

Tuberculosis (TB) continues to be a major public health problem, with a third of the world's population infected by the causative agent. In 2010, the World Health Organisation (WHO) estimated that about 9 million first episodes of TB and an additional 1.2 million subsequent cases occurred in patients with at least one previous episode while approximately 1.5 million deaths due to TB occurred worldwide.[1]

Social factors recognised to be driving the increase in TB globally include overcrowding resulting from urbanisation, neglect by national programmes, late reporting, non-compliance to treatment regime as well as stigma associated with the disease.[2] Suspected patients do not report at hospitals/clinics for early diagnosis and treatment because of the fear of being stigmatized, although these services are largely free. For instance, in Ghana, the *Akan* term/name for TB is *nsamanwa*, meaning "ghost cough", a clear indication that once you are suspected to be suffering from TB, you are regarded as dead or a ghost.[3,4] Thus, TB is equated with death sentence, a situation which encourages the concealment of the condition.

Africa, home to 11% of the world's population, carries 29% of the global burden of tuberculosis cases and 34% of related deaths. WHO estimated that close to 50,000 new TB cases occurred in 2007 in Ghana, making it the 19th among African countries most burdened with TB.[5] The main strategy being used for the control of this disease, Directly Observed Treatment Short Course (DOTS), is based on case detection and antimycobacterial treatment for at least six months using multiple drugs. In Ghana the treatment regimen consists of a two-month intensive phase (daily intake of isoniazid, rifampicin, ethambutol and pyrazinamide) and a four-month continuous phase comprising daily intake of isoniazid and rifampicin. This approach allows patients to take their daily medication under observation, thereby improving treatment compliance. Central to this control strategy is microbiological (laboratory) confirmation of clinical diagnosis before start of treatment and for monitoring response to treatment in order to declare a TB patient cured. The main method in use currently, especially in low-income countries, is microscopic detection of acid-fast bacilli in sputum. This method is cheap, rapid and does not demand elaborate infrastructure and expertise. However, it lacks specificity and sensitivity (detecting about 50% of cases), cannot determine the drug susceptibility status of the infecting strain, can also be subjective if not quality controlled and, above all, it was developed over a century ago.

In addition to issues associated with microscopy, a major challenge to the DOTS strategy in TB control globally is the incidence of strains of the causative agent resistant to the first line anti-TB drugs, especially rifampicin (RIF) and isoniazid (INH). Individuals infected by such strains are not able to be cured by the DOTS treatment strategy and also make case management more complicated and expensive. There are an estimated 460,000 multi-drug resistant TB (MDR-TB) cases reported each year and approximately 25,000 of these cases are expected to have extensively drug-resistant TB (XDRTB). MDR-TB requires 18-24 months of treatment with expensive second-line drugs, some of which are injectable agents. The cure rate is much lower than for drug susceptible TB, only around 60%. Adding to the problem of drug-resistant TB is that no new anti-TB drug has been licensed since the discovery of ethambutol in the 1960s.

## The causative agent

Tuberculosis is caused by a group of closely related gram positive bacteria, together referred to as the *Mycobacterium tuberculosis* complex (MTBC).[6] Even though genetically these species are quite close they have varying host specificity: *Mycobacterium tuberculosis* (MTB) and *Mycobacterium africanum* (MAF) are the main causative agents of TB in humans though *Mycobacterium canettii* (MCT) has occasionally been identified in TB cases from the Horn of Africa, whereas *Mycobacterium bovis* is primarily a pathogen of cattle,[7,8] *Mycobacterium microti* a pathogen of voles,[2,9] *Mycobacterium caprae* a pathogen of goats[10] and *Mycobacterium pinnipedii* a pathogen of seals and sea lions.[11] While *Mycobacterium tuberculosis* is globally distributed, *M. africanum* has a limited geographical distribution, found only in West Africa, from Senegal to Cameroon (Figure 10.1).[12]

Potential solutions to the problems associated with TB control include the development of new tools such as simple but sensitive diagnostic tools that detect the drug-resistance status of the infecting strain, rational design of new drugs and an effective TB vaccine. The Noguchi Memorial Institute for Medical Research (NMIMR) in collaboration with other research partners, is contributing to the global fight against TB by conducting studies that aim to improve understanding of disease epidemiology, genetic diversity within the causative agent, elucidation of biomarkers and laboratory diagnosis. This chapter addresses these issues in the following related sub-sections. Section one presents the role of stigma in low case detection and treatment in Sissala East District, sections two and three look at genomic diversity and drug resistance within the causative agent respectively.

## 1. The role of stigma in low case detection and treatment of TB in Sissala East District

### Introduction

The burden of TB is greatest in developing countries, which account for about 95% of TB patients.[1] In Ghana, tuberculosis remains a serious cause of preventable adult morbidity and mortality.[13] Health-related stigma is characterised by social disqualification of individuals and populations who are identified with particular health problems.[14] The Akan name *nsamanwa,* which literally means "ghost cough", connotes death and fear.[13,15] Stigma may serve as a significant barrier to case finding and treatment.[16] The objective of this study was to understand local features of TB and why virtually no new cases were being reported from the Sissala East District, for more than 5 years.

# Approach

The study was conducted in the Sissala East District which had a population of about 56,528 in 2010.[17] Tumu is the district capital and the people are mainly farmers. The study was descriptive, employing qualitative and quantitative methods for data collection. Six (three female groups) focus group discussions (FGD) were held with adults (18 years and above). In-depth interviews (IDI) were conducted with three chiefs, three queenmothers/women representatives, six health workers and eight traditional healers. The qualitative data helped to determine the ethnographic features of TB in the district. Insider perspective (emic) interviews, instruments used for assessing representations of illness or specified health problems from the insiders' perspective, were conducted with 61 persons with persistent cough for more than 14 days. These persons were expediently selected by adopting the snowball technique for sample selection. Emic blends qualitative and quantitative approaches to study illness-related experience, meaning and behaviour.[18] Qualitative data were analysed with MaxQda software to perform content analysis thematically. Quantitative data were analysed in EpiInfo version 3.3.2 to generate descriptive statistics for presentation.

## Results and Discussion

Persistent cough was recognized as a major health problem in Tumu and there are local names for it. Most (85.2%) people called it *Kesibine/kesibelle*. Others names were: *Kukuezine*, *Kesepagpon*, *Boye* and *Kesidengdeng*. All these names have to do with either persistent cough or coughing with blood.

### Causes

The people were aware of how TB is transmitted but also had some misconceptions about how the disease is caused, as shown in the narratives below.

*...when you sit nearer to somebody who is coughing and you breathe in his or her cough, you will get it* (Female opinion leader, IDI).

*...When you step on an infected person's saliva, you will be infected too* (Ladies, FGD).

...*kessibine is transmitted through sexual intercourse with an infected person ...drinking fresh milk from infected cow could also cause it* (Male opinion leader, IDI).

...*the disease is transmitted through exchange of saliva with an infected person ...through the sharing of handkerchief with an infected person. It is also caused during sexual intercourse, especially when the woman coughs during the act...* (Male, FGD).

Generally, respondents were aware of how TB is transmitted. They however have strong local beliefs about how one can be infected with TB. These misconceptions were no different from other studies[16] and there is a need for education to disabuse the minds of the people about the causes of TB.

## Gender difference

Most respondents (80.3%) said TB affects women more than men. These gender differences were seen mostly in the distress suffered by female suspected TB patients as captured in the following narratives:

...*there are differences, the truth is that women with suspected TB find it difficult to live with the disease, for instance, a woman with TB will not get a husband but a man with TB can get a wife. ...people relate differently to male and female TB patients ...no one will suspect a man with TB as having AIDS but every woman with TB is suspected of having AIDS and this makes life more difficult for women with TB than men* (Ladies, FGD)

...*I know that women suffer for having all diseases than men(sic) and TB is just one of them ...a man with prolong (sic) cough can marry and do all sorts of things but this was not the case for women, they cannot find husbands and those who were married could suffer divorce or neglect...* (Men, FGD).

## Stigma

Majority (63.9%) of those with persistent cough said they had never consciously tried to prevent others from knowing that they were coughing. However, 29.5% of them said they have tried to hide their condition from others. Reasons for attempted concealment were presented as follows:

*...TB is viewed in this community as bad and dangerous, so if you have it, people will not want to associate with you ...they will not want to eat with you, this makes you feel uncomfortable wherever you are...* (Ladies, FGD).

When respondents with no persistent cough were asked "how will you relate to your partner should he/she have TB?," the following narratives represented their responses;

*...I will not eat with her or eat any leftover from her plate ...I will not have sex with her and will not share a drinking cup with her, though I will support her to attend clinic for treatment* (Men, FGD).

*...I will relate nicely with him but will not eat with him ...it is not good to get closer to him* (Ladies, FGD).

Majority (70.5%) of suspected persons interviewed said the condition makes them think less of themselves, feel shame and feel less respected in the community.

*...once people know that you have TB, they will not want to have anything to do with you. They will look at you as a good for nothing person who is awaiting death; they think less of you, especially when they think that you got the disease through sexual pollution* (Ladies, FGD)

It became clear that women bear the brunt of TB related distresses though globally, it is known that men suffer more from TB than women.[1] Could it be that women are reluctant to report for diagnosis? This is a question that TB control programmes must seek to answer. TB-related stigma, especially directed at women, was high in the district and this calls for stigma reduction interventions like mobilizing patients to receive treatment in the community with the support and involvement of community leaders, care providers and traditional healers. This should be accompanied by educational messages that emphasize the point that TB is not deadly once patients are on effective treatment available at health facilities. The need for patients to complete their treatment should also be emphasized.

## Case detection and treatment

There was no capacity at the sub-district facilities to test suspected TB cases. This was causing delay in getting patients into treatment. Currently, samples are sent to Tumu district hospital for testing and results are either not sent back or sent after a long wait.

*...this girl (pointing to the girl); ...it took more than one year to get her into treatment ...the first sample we sent Tumu, it took more than three months to be told that it was negative but the girl was still coughing seriously ...the school teachers brought her back to the clinic several times, so I took another sample ...as for that one, we never heard about it... About three months ago, I sent a third sample ...followed it up every market day until about two weeks ago... the result came and it was positive. ...now she is on medication and looking better now. How can you explain this to the patient? ...how can you ask them to keep coming to you...?* (A nurse in charge of a sub-district facility, IDI)

Traditional healers were treating TB with local medications but were willing to collaborate with the control programme to improve access to biomedical treatment.

*...I am willing to help the control programme to identify and deliver medications (sic) to TB patients in my community, what I need is respect* (Traditional healer, IDI).

Traditional healers were aware of treatment default as captured in the following:

*...some people naturally do not like taking medicine and must be supervised to take it, for such people, once their condition gets better they stop taking the medication* (Traditional healer, IDI).

Communication between peripheral facilities and the district laboratory should be improved to help sub-district staff make early clinical decisions regarding infection status of suspected cases. This will reduce the delay between the time the patient is seen and sample taken and the time he/she gets into treatment. Laboratory technicians must be made to know the importance of their work in saving lives. The use of mobile phones (voice or text message) to communicate laboratory results to sub-district facilities should be considered in order to enhance communication.

## Conclusion

People's understanding of TB as a deadly disease should be an entry point to encourage appropriate treatment behaviour by emphasising that TB becomes deadly only when not treated at the clinic/hospital early. The willingness of traditional healers to collaborate with the control programme should be explored; they could become community-based case finders. To do this, they must be trained and given clearly defined roles to refer suspected patients to the clinic early. Useful knowledge on transmission must be emphasized in any health education programmes in the district since it will otherwise be difficult to change local beliefs.

## 2. Understanding the genomic diversity within *Mycobacterium tuberculosis* complex (MTBC) Isolates from Ghana

### Introduction

The species of the MTBC exhibit low DNA sequence diversity, a trait the MTBC share with other deadly bacterial pathogens, including the causative agents of leprosy, anthrax and plague, as such they are said to be genetically monomorphic.[19] Consequently, the general dogma was that genetic diversity within the MTBC is negligible and has no phenotypic consequence, such as host pathogen interaction which affects the ability to produce successful infection, propensity to develop drug resistance, transmission and antigenic variation which could have implication for the universal application of control tools like vaccine or diagnostics.[20,21] With current advances in molecular biology, we now know that the MTBC exhibit a clear bio-geographical population structure, underscoring the importance for genetic diversity studies to be conducted in different geographical areas, and that genomic diversity is important and could have an effect on disease epidemiology.[22,23,24] This section describes how NMIMR is using the techniques of DNA fingerprinting to examine the molecular diversity of the different circulating *Mycobacterium tuberculosis* complex strains in Ghana.

### Approach

Isolates: Mycobacterial species were isolated from patients presenting at various health facilities in Ghana with sputum-positive pulmonary tuberculosis. Sputum specimens after decontamination were cultured in duplicate on two Lowenstein-Jensen slopes, one supplemented with glycerol and the other with 0.4% sodium pyruvate to enhance the isolation of *M. africanum* and *M. bovis*. The isolates were first confirmed as acid-fast bacilli using Ziehl–Neelsen staining.

Genotyping: After DNA extraction, the MTBC were confirmed by polymerase chain reaction (PCR) indicating the presence of the insertion sequence IS*6110* and rpoβ gene. Species were defined by analysing for large sequence polymorphisms (LSP) at the regions of difference (RD) 9, 12 and 4 using published flanking primers and sub/lineage classification were done with lineage specific single nucleotide polymorphisms (SNPs) by real-time PCR according to the Taqman protocol. All isolates that were confirmed as MTBC were further typed by spoligotyping as previously described.[25,26] Briefly, the direct repeat region of each genome was amplified using primers DRa (59-CCG AGA GGG GAC GGA AAC-39) and biotinylated Drb (59-GGT TTT GGG TCT GAC GAC-39). The amplified DNA was tested for the presence or absence of the 43 specific spacers by hybridization with a set of 43 oligonucleotides immobilised on cellulose acetate paper. Clustering was determined by mycobacterial interspersed repetitive unit-variable number tandem ascot (MIRM-VNTR) typing.

## Results and Discussion

### Strain typing and lineage identification

We were able to establish in our laboratory modern methods including spoligotyping, large sequence polymorphism analysis, allele-specific PCR and other PCR-based tools for characterisation of *Mycobacterium* spp. In order to study genotype-phenotype associations, phylogenetically robust molecular markers and appropriate genotyping tools are required. We therefore established, in addition to the methods indicated above, real-time a PCR-based, SNP typing protocol for genotyping isolates collected over a period of four years. We found that 80% of the species causing TB was *Mycobacterium tuberculosis* **sensu stricto (MTBss)** and the remaining 20% were classified as *Mycobacterium africanum*; no *M. bovis* was detected. There is a perception that the importance of *M. africanum* in West Africa is declining and with the increase in population density, the seemingly more virulent *M. tuberculosis* will eliminate *M. africanum*. This perception can further reduce the little attention being paid to *M. africanum*. Our findings, however, stress the importance of *Mycobacterium africanum* as an important pathogen in Ghana and defeats the perception that *M. africanum* prevalence is declining in West Africa and that *M. africanum* is still present in Ghana at almost the same prevalence rate (about 20%) as previously reported.[27]

The outcomes of TB infections in humans are extremely variable, ranging from lifelong latent infection to active disease with variable degrees of extra-pulmonary involvement. At the same time, it is well established that the outcome of infection is the result of cross-talk between the host and the pathogen, which in the pathogen is determined by the genetic background of the infecting strain. Early studies using animal models and macrophage cell line studies indicate that the place of isolation influences the virulence and immuno-genicity within the MTBC lineages.[13,28] In addition, studies conducted by de Jong *et al.* suggest that *M. africanum* is less virulent than *M. tuberculosis sensu stricto*, since a study in The Gambia demonstrated that although *M. tuberculosis sensu stricto* and *M. africanum* infected cases were equally able to transmit infections to household contacts, more contacts infected with MTBss progressed to active disease.[13] Furthermore, findings from the work of this group also indicate that the main human MTBCs may differ in gene expression which will have influence on design and efficacy of control tools such as vaccine, drugs and diagnostics. Our findings point out that for the testing of new control tools, Ghana is one of the few countries which harbour both lineages of *M. africanum* (i.e. West Africa I and West Africa II) and *M. tuberculosis sensu stricto*.

In addition, the fact that *M. africanum* can be continuously detected in about 20% of TB cases demonstrates that *M. africanum* is successful within the West African population and the reason for this needs to be further investigated.

## Molecular epidemiology: prevalence and distribution of various sub-lineages and strains

Six hundred and thirteen isolates have been spoligotyped (508 (82.87%) M. tuberculosis and 105 (17.13%) M. africanum) and from these isolates 118 different spoligotypes were identified: 81 patterns for M. tuberculosis and 37 patterns for M. africanum. Four hundred and seventy-five of the 508 (93.5%) M. tuberculosis isolates clustered within 47 different spoligotypes, compared to 81/108 (77.1%) of the M. africanum isolates grouped in 13 spoligotyping clusters (OR: 2.78, 95% CI = 1.00–7.35, p = 0.02). Among the remaining 58 non-clustered isolates 18 had previously defined shared Spoligotype numbers. Twenty-two of the remaining orphan strains (not previously identified and not in a cluster) were M. africanum

The main sub-lineage found within the M. tuberculosis by spoligotyping include the Cameroon sub-lineage, which has also been found to be prevalent in Cameroon and accounted for 50% of all the isolates. The Cameroon family has also been identified in other West African countries.[23,29] We therefore hypothesise that this family could have been the first sub-lineage within the Euro-American lineage to establish itself, thus being the most dominant M. tuberculosis strain found across West Africa. In addition to these, other sub-lineages of M. tuberculosis strains identified in Ghana included the famous Beijing genotype found mainly in South-East Asia, and implicated in a number of disease outbreaks and occurrence of resistant disease and lineages like EAI and Delhi/CASI. The continual identification of the Beijing sub-lineage, which is associated with drug resistance and disease outbreaks in other parts of the world, is of concern as it could influence the trend in control of TB in Ghana. We found that M. tuberculosis isolates were more likely than the M. africanum isolates to be part of a spoligotyping cluster. This observation could indicate an overall higher genetic diversity among M. africanum compared to M. tuberculosis in Ghana. This supports the hypothesis that M. africanum established itself in West Africa before the Euro-American M. tuberculosis lineage was introduced during European exploration and colonization. Alternatively, M. tuberculosis might be more transmissible than M. africanum in Ghana. However, whether these spoligotyping clusters represent linked transmission events will need to be confirmed by genotyping methods such as MIRU-VNTR which exhibit a higher discriminatory power.

While the established methods (e.g. spoligotyping and SNP) have been useful in understanding the circulating strains in Ghana relative to that of other parts of the world, they are incapable of being used for detailed micro-epidemiological studies, which are good for information on factors enhancing the extent of disease spread across the country. We thus have established a more robust PCR method, a customised MIRU-VNTR that is specific to the main lineages found in Ghana. This technique was based on earlier *in silico* analysis that found that not all the loci within the standard 24 loci MIRU-VNTR are discriminatory with respect to distinct lineages.[30] Therefore, only the 12 most discriminatory loci for a specific sub/lineage among the 24 loci MIRU-VNTR was used for characterisation. To establish the method, we evaluated the 12 customized loci which is lineage specific against the standard method to determine the discriminatory power between the two methods and the most discriminatory loci which could further reduce the number of loci used for the assay. Preliminary findings from the study give credence to the lineage specific customized assay. This finding will reduce the cost and time involved in transmission dynamics studies within TB control.

More males reported with TB than females from all the health facilities studies. Approximately two thirds of the participants (66%) were males and this compares very well with other reports.[31] The reasons why more men report with TB than women cannot be explained. However, as indicated in the earlier section of this chapter, women are more stigmatised than men and this could account for a lower reporting rate among women. It could be that women do not have time to go for treatment or they hide their condition due to fear of being stigmatized or they do not have the final decision on when and where to seek help and therefore do not access treatment. It could also simply be that males engage in more TB risk-related activities, hence are prone to the disease.

# 3. Defining the molecular basis of drug resistance within the MTBC

## Introduction

The conventional method for determining drug susceptibility of TB strains is slow and can take about three months to get results, making it unsuitable for case management. This section describes how we have established a commercial assay MTBDR*plus* (Hain Lifescience, Nehren, Germany) and used it to analyse set of strains and are using it to support the National TB Control Programme (NTP) in case management. The design of these kits was based on earlier sequencing analysis that determined mutations associated with drug resistance. However, such studies were done using strains collected in countries where the Euro-American lineage dominates. At the same time there is evidence that the genetic background of a pathogen affects the type and propensity to mutate. Taking into consideration that the distribution of human MTBC lineages is geographically linked, it is crucial for mutational studies in different geographical regions to see the applicability of the rapid diagnostic kits in diagnosis of drug resistance. Hence, this section also describes drug resistance survey by conventional and molecular methods, including sequencing of drug targets of isolates collected from Ghana for mutational studies.

## Approach

### Drug resistance analysis

The indirect proportion method was used to determine the susceptibility pattern of mycobacterial isolates to isoniazid (INH; 0.2 mg/ml), rifampicin (RIF; 40 mg/ml), streptomycin (STR; 4 mg/ml), and ethambutol (EMB; 2 mg/ml) by cultivating on Lowenstein Jensen medium. In addition the susceptibility of the isolates to INH and RIF was determined by using the MTBDR*plus* DNA-based detection method. The results of both assays were interpreted as drug sensitive or resistant. The drug targets of isolates found to be resistant to distinct drugs were then sequenced and the sequences obtained compared against that of the *M. tuberculosis* reference strain $H_{37}Rv$ from the tuberculist database using the Staden R software.

## Results and Discussion

The drug susceptibility patterns of 122 *Mycobacterium tuberculosis* and *M. africnum* isolates were tested using the proportion method. We found that the *M. tuberculosis* isolates are more likely to develop any form of drug resistance when compared to all *M. africanum* (OR = 2.74, CI 95 % 1.01–8.24, p=0.03). This observation was mainly driven by the differences in resistance to STR. This observation goes on to indicate that strain genetic background influences the occurrence of drug resistance and probably the conferring of mutations.[32]

Four hundred and eighty-seven clinical MTBC isolates (411 *M. tuberculosis* and 76 *M. africanum*), mainly from pulmonary tuberculosis patients receiving care in health facilities across southern Ghana were analysed by the MTBDR*plus* assay (Table 1). Thirty-nine (8.00%) of them were resistant to INH, 20 (4.10%) to RIF; mono-resistance to RIF and INH was found to be 13 (2.67%) and 32 (6.57%) respectively. Defining multi-drug resistant TB (MDR) as resistance to at least INH and RIF, 7 (1.44%) MDR isolates were identified while 52 (10.68%) isolates had some form of drug resistance. As indicated in Table 1, we did not find statistical support to indicate that the propensity to mutate or to develop drug resistance to INH and RIF varies between the two pathogens. However, *M. tuberculosis* isolates were more resistant in all criteria used for analysis. All 13 isolates that were mono-resistant to RIF were *M. tuberculosis*. A larger sample size may be needed in a future study to look into associations between *M. tuberculosis* and *M. africanum*. This objective will be explored in an ongoing study funded by the Wellcome Trust.

Table 10.1: Distribution of drug resistance detected by MTBDR*plus* assay

| Drug Tested | M. tuberculosis (n=411) N (%) | M. africanum (n=76) N (%) | p value |
|---|---|---|---|
| INH | 33 (8.03%) | 6 (7.89%) | 0.85 |

**Table 10.1: (continued)   Distribution of drug resistance detected by
MTBDRplus assay continued**

| RIF | 19 (4.62%) | 1 (1.32%) | 0.309 |
|-----|-----------|-----------|-------|
| MDR | 6 (1.46%) | 1 (1.32%) | 0.667 |
| Any | 46 (11.19%) | 6 (7.89%) | 0.513 |

To characterise drug resistance associated mutations from Ghana, 32 phenotypic INH resistant and RIF resistant isolates were analysed. Three genomic loci; *inhApro* (promotor region of the gene encoding the 3-oxoacyl-[acyl-carrier protein] reductase), *katG* (the gene encoding catalase-peroxidase-peroxynitritase T which, apart from hydrolysis of peroxides, also activates isoniazid into the active drug) and *ahpC* (gene encoding the alkyl hydroperoxide reductase sub C, also involved with destruction of peroxides but does not activate isoniazid and has been linked with INH resistance) were amplified and sequenced. The sequence analyses identified 4 different mutations (-8T/C, -15C/T, -42G/C or -102G/C) in the *inhApro* in 7 isolates. Two of these mutations (-42G/C and -102G/C) however, were novel mutations. Twenty-one of the INH-resistant isolates had the most commonly reported mutation (S315T) in the katG locus and one isolate had an additional mutation (I317V) within the same locus which has not been reported before. No mutation was seen in the ahpC locus. Four different mutations (D435V, H445D, H445Y and S450L) were identified among the RIF resistant isolates and all four were located within the 81bp hotspot region of the rpoβ.

Even though TB is treatable, its control has been hampered by the emergence of drug resistant (DR) TB bacilli.[33] The steady increase in the frequency of DR-TB has drawn worldwide attention to understanding the molecular basis of drug resistant TB because better knowledge of the molecular mechanisms involved is useful for rapid detection and will also promote the search for new targets for drug activity and drug development.[34,35]

From the MTBDR*plus* assay, 39 isolates representing 8.01% of the total were resistant to INH (mono resistant and MDR) as compared to 20 isolates representing 4.11% that were resistant to RIF (*p=0.016*), which may support the assertion that INH resistance facilitates resistance to other drugs.[36] DNA sequence analyses of INH and RIF target genes detected mainly known mutations, with the exception of three mutations; -47G/C and -102G/C in *inhApro* and I317V in *katG* which have not been reported and further research is required to ascertain whether they contribute to drug resistance or they are just random mutations. If they are resistant-conferring mutations, then it will reduce the sensitivity of current WHO-recommended rapid diagnostics such as MTBDR*plus* in Ghana. On the other hand, all mutations detected in *katG* gene which lead to high-level INH resistance are known and are in-use for the rapid diagnosis of INH resistance.[37] Likewise, all mutations identified within the rpoβ gene -D435V, H445D and H445Y[38] and S450L[39,40] are known. The National Tuberculosis Programme with the support of the NMIMR, has established the MTBDR*plus* assay to support treatment of TB patients in Ghana. Findings from this study are very important as they put more confidence in the diagnostic value of the MTBDR*plus* assay for the support of TB case management in Ghana.

## Conclusions

Our work on tuberculosis in the past years indicates that *M. africanum* is still present in Ghana at almost the same prevalence rate (20%) as previously reported[13] and within the regions that we worked in, MAF is uniformly distributed. We also found that there seem to be differences in the propensity to develop DR-TB and that there may be different drug-conferring mutations in some Ghanaian MTBC isolates, which has implications for the sensitivity/specificity of the World Health Organisation-approved rapid kits for the management of drug resistance cases. Additional works are needed to understand the comprehensive genetic diversity between and among these lineages and sub-lineages of MTBC. Under new funding schemes, we are looking at:

- Urban and rural effects on distribution of members of MTBCs and risk factors for transmission;
- Comparing the transmission of MTB and MAF and associated risk factors, such as HIV, DR, diabetes in these areas;
- Comparative whole-genome sequencing analysis which will give a comprehensive picture of the variation and the evolutionary

forces shaping diversity in Ghanaian MTBC strains and its effects on differential gene expression;

• Characterise the immune response of individuals infected by M. tuberculosis and M. africanum to some antigens before and over the course of anti-TB therapy in order to provide new insights into host-pathogen interactions in tuberculosis (TB), and to identify a putative biomarker for TB treatment outcome and cure.

Findings from these ongoing studies will provide useful information for new antigens for both diagnostics and vaccine development as well as targets for new drug design. The differences in drug resistance-conferring mutations will be known, which will have implications for the application of the current molecular-based drug susceptibility assays recently endorsed by WHO.

## Acknowledgements

We would like to thank our collaborators, especially the National Tuberculosis Control Programme (NTCP) of Ghana and Prof. Sebastien Gagneux of Switzerland. We received funding from the Leverhulme-Royal Society Africa Award, the Wellcome Trust grant number 097134/Z/11/Z and UNICEF/UNDP/World Bank/WHO Special Programme for Research and Training in Tropical Diseases (TDR) and the NTCP of Ghana.

## References

1.  World Health Organization. Global TB Control Report. 2011; Geneva: World Health Organization.
2.  Hargreaves, J. R., Boccia, D., Evans, C. A., Adato, M., Petticrew, M. and Porter, D.H. The social determinants of tuberculosis: from evidence to action. *Am J Public Health* 2010; 101: 654-662.
3.  Ghana Health Service. Technical, Policy and Guidelines for TB/HIV Collaboration in Ghana. 2006. Accra: Ghana Health Service.
4.  Ghana Health Service. Report--*Health Programmes*. 2008. Accra: GHS.
5.  World Health Organization Global. *TB Report.* 2009. Geneva: World Health Organization.

6.   Comas, I, and Gagneux S. A role for systems epidemiology in tuberculosis research. *Trend Microbiol* 2011; 19 (10): 492-500.
7.   Smith, T. A. Comparative studies of bovine tubercle bacilli and of human bacilli from sputum. *J Exp Med* 1898; 3: 451–511.
8.   Garnier, T., Eiglmeier, K., Camus, J.C., Medina, N., Mansoor, H. *et al.* The complete genome sequence of *Mycobacterium bovis. Proc Natl Acad Sci* USA. 2003; 100: 7877-7882.
9.   Frota, C.C., Hunt, D.M., Buxton, R.S., Rickman, L., Hinds, J. *et al.* Genome structure in the vole bacillus, *Mycobacterium microti*, a member of the *Mycobacterium tuberculosis* complex with a low virulence for humans. *Microbiol* 2004; 150: 1519-1527.
10.  Hershberg, R., Lipatov, M., Small, P. M., Sheffer, H., Niemann, S. *et al.* High functional diversity in *Mycobacterium tuberculosis* driven by genetic drift and human demography. *PLoS Biol* 2008; 6 e311. doi:10.1371/ Journal. *PLoS Biol*.0060311.
11.  Aranaz, A., Cousins, D., Mateos, A., Dominguez, L. Elevation of *Mycobacterium tuberculosis* subsp.caprae Aranaz *et al.* 1999 to species rank as *Mycobacterium caprae* comb. nov., sp. Nov. *Int J Syst Evol Microbiol* 2003; 53: 1785-1789
12.  Cousins, D. V., Bastida, R., Cataldi, A., Quse, V., Redrobe, S. *et al.* Tuberculosis in seals caused by a novel member of the *Mycobacterium tuberculosis* complex: *Mycobacterium pinnipedii* sp. nov. *Int J Syst Evol Microbiol* 2003; 53: 1305-1314.
13.  de Jong, B. C., Anthonio, M., Gagneux, S. *Mycobacterium africanum* - Review of an important cause of human tuberculosis in West Africa. *PLoS Negl Trop Dis* 2010; 4: e744.
14.  Lawn, S. D., Achempong, J. V. V. Pulmonary tuberculosis in adults: factors associated with mortality at a Ghanaian teaching hospital. *West Afr J Med* 1999; 18: 270-274.
15.  Goffman, E. Stigma: Notes on the management of spoiled identity. 1963. Englewood Cliffs: Prentice Hall.
16.  Lawn, S. D. Tuberculosis in Ghana: social stigma and compliance with treatment. *Int J Tuberc Lung Dis* 2000; 4: 1190-1191.
17.  Weiss, M. G., Ramakrishna, J., Somma, D. Health-related stigma: Rethinking concepts and interventions. *Psychol Health Med* 2006; 11: 277-287.
18.  Ghana Statistical Service. (2010). Population and Housing Census; summary of final results. Accra: GSS, May 2012.
19.  Weiss, M. G. Cultural epidemiology: an introduction and overview. *Anthropol Med* 2001; 8: 5-29.

20. Achtman, M. Evolution, population structure, and phylogeography of genetically monomorphic bacterial pathogens. *Ann Rev Microbiol* 2008; 62: 53-70.

21. Brosch, R., Gordon, S. V., Pym, A., Eiglmeier, K., Garnier. T. *et al.* Comparative genomics of the mycobacteria. *Int J. Med Microbiol* 2000; 290: 143-152.

22. Supply, P., Warren, R. M., Banuls, A-L., Lesjean, S., van der Spuy, G.D. *et al.* Linkage disequilibrium between minisatellite loci supports clonal evolution of *Mycobacterium tuberculosis* in a high tuberculosis incidence area. *Mol Microbiol* 2003; 47: 529-538.

23. Ozcaglar, C., Shabbeer, A., Vandenberg, S., Yerner, B., Bennett, K. P. Sublineage structure analysis of *Mycobacterium tuberculosis* complex strains using multiple-biomarker tensors. *BMC Genomics* 2011; 12 (suppl 2: S1.) doi: 10.1186/1471-2164-12-S2-S1.

24. Yeboah-Manu, D., Asante-Poku, A., Bodmer, T., Stucki, D., Koram, K. *et al.* Genotypic diversity and drug susceptibility patterns among *M. tuberculosis*complex isolates from South-western Ghana. *PLoS ONE* 2011; 6(7): e21906. doi:10.1371/journal.pone. 0021906.

25. Gagneux, S. Host-pathogen coevolution in human tuberculosis. *Phil Trans R Soc* 2012; 367: 850-859.

26. Ferdinand, S., Valetudie, G., Sola, C., Rastogi, N. Data mining of *Mycobacterium tuberculosis* complex genotyping results using mycobacterial interspersed repetitive units validates the clonal structure of spoligotyping-defined families. *Res Microbiol*; 2004; 155: 647–654.

27. Brudey, K., Driscoll, J. R., Rigout, L., Prodinger, W. M., Gori, A. *et al.* *Mycobacterium tuberculosis* complex genetic diversity: mining the fourth international spoligotyping database (SpolDB4) for classification, population genetics and epidemiology. *BMC Microbiol* 2006; 6: 23.

28. Mitchison, D .A., Wallace, J. G., Bhatia, A. L., Selkon, J. B., Subbaiah,T. V. *et al.* . A comparison of the virulence in guinea-pigs of South Indian and British tubercle bacilli. *Tubercle*; 1960; 41:1-22. [PubMed: 14423002].

29. McEvoy, C.R.E., Cloete, R., Muller, B., Schurch, A.C., van Helden, P.D. *et al.* Comparative analysis of *Mycobacterium tuberculosis* pe and ppe genes reveals high sequence variation and an apparent absence of selective constraints. *PLoS ONE* 2012; 7(4): e30593. doi:10.1371/journal. pone.0030593.

30. de Jong, B. C., Hill, P. C., Aiken, A., Awine, T., Antonio, M. *et al.* Progression to active tuberculosis, but not transmission, varies by

*Mycobacterium tuberculosis* lineage in The Gambia. *J Infect Dis* 2008; 198: 1–7.

31. Cadmus, S., Hill, V., van Soolingen, D., Rastogi., N. Spoligotype profile of *Mycobacterium tuberculosis* complex strains from HIV-positive and negative patients in Nigeria: a comparative analysis. *J Clin Microbiol* 2011; 49(1): 220-226.

32. Comas, I., Homolka, S., Niemann, S., Gagneux, S. Genotyping of genetically monomorphic bacteria: DNA sequencing in *Mycobacterium tuberculosis* highlights the limitations of current methodologies. *PLoS ONE*; 2009; 4(11): e7815. doi:10.1371/journal.pone.0007815.

33. Yeboah-Manu, D., Asante-Poku, A., Assan Ampah, K., Kpeli, G., Danso, E.*et al.* Drug susceptibility pattern of *Mycobacterium tuberculosis* isolates from Ghana; correlation with clinical response. *Mycobact Dis* 2012; 2: 107. doi:10.4172/2161-1068.1000107.

34. Perkins, M. D., Cunningham, J. Facing the Crisis: improving the diagnosis of tuberculosis in the HIV era. *J Inf Dis* 2007; 196(S1): S15-S27.

35. Udwadia, Z. Emergence of new forms of totally drug-resistant tuberculosis bacilli, *Chest*, April 6 2009 http://chestjournal.chestpubs.org. Accessed January 2013

36. World Health Organization. '*Totally Drug Resistant*' *Tuberculosis*: WHO consultation on the diagnostic definition and treatment options', Geneva: World Health Organization, 2012 www.who.int/tb/challenges/xdr.

37. Bergval, I., Sengstake, S., Brankova, N., Levterova, V., Abadía, E. *et al.* Combined species identification, genotyping, and drug resistance detection of *Mycobacterium tuberculosis* cultures by MLPA on a bead-based array. *PLoS ONE* 2012; 7(8): e43240. doi:10.1371/ journal. pone.0043240.

38. Brossier, F. N., Veziris, C., Truffot-Pernot, V., Jarlier., Sougakoff, W. Performance of the genotype MTBDR line probe assay for detection of resistance to rifampin and isoniazid in strains of *Mycobacterium tuberculosis* with low- and high-level resistance. *J Clin Microbiol* 2006; 44: 3659-3664.

39. Kapur, V., Whittam, T. S., Musser, J. M. Is *Mycobacterium tuberculosis* 15,000 years old? *J Infect Dis* 1994; 170: 1348–1389.

40. Donnabella, V., Martiniuk, F., Kinney, D.,Bacerdo, M., Bonk, S. *et al.* Isolation of the gene for the beta subunit of RNA polymerase from rifampicin-resistant *Mycobacterium tuberculosis* and identification of new mutations. *Am J Respir Cell Mol Biol* 1994; 11(6):639-643.

# Chapter 11
## Studies to Improve The Understanding of Buruli Ulcer Transmission

Anthony Ablordey, Nana Ama Amissah, Innocent Afeke,
Alfred Dodoo, Dorothy Yeboah Manu and Phyllis Addo

## Introduction

Buruli ulcer (BU), caused by infection with Mycobacterium ulcerans, is a necrotising skin disease reported in over 34 countries worldwide but mainly a public health problem in several rural sub-Saharan African communities.[1] The disease often permanently deforms its victims and is associated with huge economic and social consequences and a significant drain on the resources of an already overstretched health delivery services. In the Amansie West District of Ghana, 83% of the district's health budget in 1994 was used by 36 patients in a population of 130,000 people.[2]

Although there are convincing data to suggest that M. ulcerans is an environmental pathogen, the exact niche of the organism as well as the route of transortation are yet to be determined.[1] Recent genomic analysis gives some indication that M. ulcerans may not be able to survive in nature as a free living organism but rather may reside inside a protozoan host where it will be protected from environmental hazards such as elevated temperature and UV light.[3] Amoeba sp. has been proposed as likely host of M. ulcerans in the environment.[4,5] However, detailed investigation of the environment to detect M. ulcerans in amoeba has not been done.

Patients' isolates have been genotyped with a plethora of methods and compared in order to decipher epidemiological links among isolates. These analyses reveal remarkable genetic monomorphism, especially among isolates originating from the same geographic area.[6-13] This apparent lack of genetic diversity as well as the difficulty in cultivating M. ulcerans from the environment represents an important hindrance to the understanding of BU transmission.[7] A high-resolution typing method will be an invaluable tool for unlocking the mysteries surrounding the reservoir and transmission routes of M. ulcerans. The development and application of such typing methods are among the research priorities of the Global Buruli Ulcer Initiative.

We have developed and tested a number of high-resolution typing methods and carried out environmental analysis in BU endemic areas to identify sources of M. ulcerans in nature and the possible route of transmission. We have also investigated whether amoeba species can harbour and possibly be involved in the transmission of M. ulcerans.

# Approach

## Development of molecular typing methods

BLAST searches was used to confirm the presence of the multicopy GC-rich sequence Mtb2 in the M. ulcerans genome, and outward directed primers based on the M. ulcerans insertion element IS2404 were designed to amplify genomic regions between these repeat elements in a collection of M. ulcerans isolates. This method is designated IS2404-Mtb2 PCR[6]. For the second method, we used the tandem repeat finder algorithm of the Department of Biomathematical Science of Mount Sinai School of Medicine (http://c3.biomath.mssm.edu/trf.html) to identify potential tandem repeat loci in M. ulcerans genome sequence. We developed specific primers using the Oligo 5.0 software (National Biosciences Inc. Plymouth, Minnesota) for the amplification of each of these targets by PCR in a collection of M. ulcerans isolates.[7] Single nucleotide polymorphisms (SNPs) were detected in a total of 74 M. ulcerans patient isolates from BU endemic areas located in the Ga West, Ga East and Akuapim South districts using the amplification refractory mutation system (ARMS) as described by Röltgen et al.[14]

## Analysis of environs of endemic areas for the detection of M. ulcerans

The study was conducted in five endemic villages; Ananekrom, Nhyieso, Serebouso, Dukusen and Bebuso and two non endemic communities, Mageda and Pataban in the Asante Akim North (AAN)

District (Figure 11.1) of Ghana for a period of 10 months. AAN is the third most endemic district in Ghana. The five endemic communities had a village-based prevalence ranging from 0.47% to 2.14% in 2006 and 2007.[15] Ananekrom has consistently reported more cases than any endemic community in Ghana.

## Environmental sampling

A total of 148 environmental samples (13 water samples, 45 detritus samples, 45 trunk biofilm, and 45 plant biofilm samples) collected from water bodies near the BU endemic (n = 117) and BU non endemic (n = 31) villages were analysed. Also 62 small mammals (36 *Praomys* spp., 10 *Mastomys* spp., five *Lemniscomys* spp., three *Lophuromys* spp., four *Crocidura* spp. and four *Mus* spp.) trapped in houses and around water bodies of Ananekrom were investigated for *M. ulcerans*. Portions of the samples were decontaminated using the oxalic acid method and used for the cultivation of *M. ulcerans* and amoeba. Template DNA for the detection of *M. ulcerans* was extracted from the samples using the modified Boom method.[16]

## *TaqMan Multiplex real-time PCR assays for* M. ulcerans *detection from environmental samples*

Two TaqMan Multiplex real-time PCR assays based on *M. ulcerans* insertion sequences IS*2404*, IS*2606* and sequence encoding the ketore-ductase B domain (KR-B) developed by Fyfe *et al.,*[17] for the specific and rapid detection of *M. ulcerans* was established in our laboratory and applied to DNA extracts of the environmental samples for the detection of this pathogen.

## Cultivation and identification of amoebae

Amoebae monolayers were seeded with suspensions of *M. ulcerans* in triplicate at an approximate multiplicity of infection of 1 (*M. ulcerans* to *A. polyphaga*) and plates were incubated at 30° C as described by Gressels *et al.*[15] Non-nutrient agar plates coated with *Escherichia coli* served as medium for amoebal growth, as described by Page.[18] Plates were incubated at 30° C and read daily under a light microscope until amoebal growth was visible. Amoeba species were identified by PCR amplification with specific primers for members of the *Vahlkampfiidae*, *Naegleria sp.* and *Acanthamoeba sp.* The PCR products were sequenced using the respective PCR primers as previously described.[19-21]

## Cultivation of extra and intra-cellular mycobacteria from environmental samples

For the cultivation of intracellular mycobacteria, samples were incubated overnight in 40 mg/mL kanamycin, to kill extra cellular mycobacteria but not eukaryotic organisms. The suspension was centrifuged for 5 minutes at 500 g and the pellet resuspended in 5 mL PBS with 0.5% SDS to lyse non-mycobacterial microorganisms. The samples were then decontaminated using the oxalic acid method and the decontaminated samples inoculated onto LJ medium and incubated at 30°C and read for 52 weeks.[15]

# Results

The IS2404-Mtb2 PCR, like previous methods, delineated *M. ulcerans* according to their geographic origins. However, it resolved for the first time the Asian type into China and Japan genotypes.[6] In our pioneering work on the use of VNTR typing on a global collection of *M. ulcerans*, we identified 17 polymorphic targets including 10 novel and seven Mycobacterial Interspersed Repetitive Unit (MIRU) targets and used these to develop VNTR-based typing for *M. ulcerans*. Our study demonstrated improvement in the level of intra-species discrimination among isolates originating from the same geographic region.[7,9, 10]

For example, four *M. ulcerans* genotypes, namely the Atlantic African, East African Nile River basin, Central African Congo River basin and a unique type found in Angola, were identified amongst the hitherto genetically conserved African isolates.[11,12] Application of the VNTR typing also led to the discrimination of the French Guiana and Surinam genotypes in Central America for the first time.[7]

The VNTR method was also used for typing 72 African *M. ulcerans* strains, including 57 from Ghana, and identified three genotypes in Ghana.[10] More importantly, there were variations in distribution of the different genotypes between the two main endemic areas, while genotype 3 strains were found only in the Ga District. Genotype 2 strains were identified only in the Amansie West District. The common allelic combination found in other African isolates (genotype 1) was rarely found in Ghana. Two of the three genotypes which were found in recent Ghanaian isolates were not found in other countries. SNP typing of a collection of M. *ulcerans* isolates from residents along the Densu River valley with BU identified 10 different SNP haplotypes within the study area.

## Detection of M. *ulcerans* in samples and amoeba cultures

Three samples (2.0%) were positive for IS*2404*, with cycle threshold (CT) values of 36.31, 38.45, and 37.95, respectively. Of the three positive samples, only the water sample from Nhyieso also tested positive for IS*2606* and KR, with a difference in CT values for the two insertion elements IS*2606* and IS*2404* i.e. $\Delta$ CT (IS*2606*-IS*2404*) value of 1.96. The CT (IS*2404*) values of the other two IS*2404*-positive samples were higher than the sample that did contain IS*2606* and KR,

One hundred and sixty-six (166) amoeba cultures were obtained from 124 different samples and seven of these were positive for IS*2404*. The IS*2404* positive amoeba cultures were isolated from BU-endemic as well as BU non-endemic communities and from different microbial habitats. None of the IS*2404*-containing amoeba cultures tested positive for IS*2606* or KR-B.

The following amoebae were identified among the IS*2404* positive cultures: Vahlkampfilae (99% identical with the V. *avara* sequence in Genbank), a close relative of V. *inornata* (92% identical with the V. *inornata* sequence in Genbank), A. *lenticulata* (T5 genotype), *Acanthamoeba* sp. T11 genotype and *Acanthamoeba* sp. T4 genotype. From 15 samples (12.2%) only intracellular mycobacteria were isolated while extracellular mycobacteria were isolated from 17 samples (13.9%) and from 32 samples (26.2%) both intra- and extracellular mycobacteria were isolated. In general, the difference between the isolation frequency of extracellular and intracellular mycobacteria was not significant ($x^2 = 0.17$, p = 0.89). The relative isolation frequency of intracellular mycobacteria did not differ between BU-endemic and non-BU endemic areas (0.77 vs. 0.68; p =0.86, $x^2$

= 0.03). The type of habitat, however, did have a significant effect on the relative occurrence of intracellular mycobacteria (p = 0.002; $x^2$ = 15.1): intracellular mycobacteria were more frequently isolated from detritus samples (relative isolation frequency of 0.95) than from biofilm samples (relative isolation frequency of 0.63; p =0.01). None of the organs of the rodents was positive for IS2404.

## Discussion

We used whole genome approaches to develop molecular typing assays for M. ulcerans and have extensively studied genetic diversity in a global collection of this pathogen. Although we were able to achieve ample resolution of previously homogenous genotypes; the level of discrimination is not high enough to discern finer epidemiological details such as tracing transmission routes or deciphering reactivation and exogenous reinfection as cause of disease recurrence.

Application of SNP typing has, however, showed some modest gains in illuminating our understanding of the distribution of M. ulcerans types. In the SNP typing, 10 different haplotypes were identified within the study area and when these haplotypes were linked to the residence of the patients, it was realized that M. ulcerans haplotypes do not spread within a short time over the entire endemic region but rather form focal transmission clusters. It was also revealed that the SNP haplotypes that dominated the upper sections of the river (Densu) differed from those that dominated the lower sections.

The research community has used the methods we have developed extensively for several purposes. Most notable is their use in confirming the presence of M. ulcerans in the environment.[22,23] For example. scientists investigating BU outbreaks in Australia have used the VNTR analysis to confirm the presence of M. ulcerans in the mosquito Aedes camptorhynchus.[22] The use of this method is, however, limited by the low bacilli load of M. ulcerans in environmental specimens. The VNTR method has also been used to identify countries in which travellers might have contracted BU disease.[24]

Detection of all three targets (IS2404, IS2606 and KR) as well as the 1.96 value obtained for the $\Delta CT$ (IS2606-IS2404) in the water sample strongly indicates the presence of M. ulcerans. Although the two biofilms samples tested positive for only IS*2404*, it is probable that they also contain *M. ulcerans* in much lower quantities as their CT (IS*2404*) values were higher than that of the water sample.

While small mammals such as possums and koalas are infected with *M. ulcerans* in the wild in Australia, BU disease has not been reported in small mammals in Africa. The detection of BU disease in animals may indicate that they are exposed to the bacteria in the environment. More studies are required to investigate BU in animals in Africa.

The successful uptake and persistence of *M. ulcerans* inside *A. polyphaga in vitro* and the higher detection frequency of IS*2404* in amoeba cultures as opposed to the crude samples from the environment lead us to speculate that amoebae may act as a host for *M. ulcerans* in natural circumstances. However, our data do not reveal a significant role for protozoa in the distribution patterns of BU disease in humans.

## Conclusion

The development and application of high-resolution typing methods has contributed to revealing genetic differences in *M. ulcerans* populations. Although the gains chalked at the moment with the use of existing methods are modest and do not allow us to discern finer epidemiological details, they still permit us to identify the distribution patterns of the different genotypes of *M. ulcerans* within a given endemic area. This information, when overlaid with patients' information or history, may likely yield useful information about how BU is transmitted.

We recorded high CT values for *M. ulcerans* targets in quantitative real-time PCR giving indication of low levels of the bacterium in the environment. We have for the first time detected IS*2404* target in amoeba cultures isolated from the environment and this enables us to suggest that the protozoa can harbour *M. ulcerans*. Intracellular survival of *M. ulcerans* in amoeba may enable the bacterium to persist in the environment. The same frequency of isolation of intracellular as from extracellular sources suggests that mycobacteria commonly infect amoeba in nature. However, the detection of *M. ulcerans* in amoeba in both endemic and non-endemic areas at similar frequencies cast doubt on the role of amoeba in BU transmission. We conclude that amoeba are potential natural hosts for *M. ulcerans*, but are uncertain of their role in the transmission of *M. ulcerans* to humans.

## Acknowledgements

We thank our collaborators Prof. François Portaels, Dr. Miriam Eddyani and Dr. Lies Durnez of the Institute of Tropical Medicine, Antwerp, Prof. Herwig Leirs of the University of Antwerp, Prof. Gerd Pluschke and Dr. Katharina Roltgen of the Swiss Tropical Institute for their diverse contribution towards the studies. Funds for the projects were provided by the Flemish Inter-University Council (VLIR), the University Development Cooperation (UOS) and the Stop Buruli Initiative supported by the UBS-Optimus Foundation.

# References

1. Asiedu, K., Scherpbier, R. W., Raviglione, M. Buruli ulcer. 2000; 1-160. WHO/CDS/GBUI/2000.1 Geneva: WHO

2. Asiedu, K., Etuaful, S. Socioeconomic implications of Buruli ulcer in Ghana: a three-year review. *Am J Trop Med Hyg* 1998; 59:1015-1022.

3. Stinear, T. P., Seemann, T., Pidot, S., Frigui, W., Reysset, G., *et al.* Reductive evolution and niche adaptation inferred from the genome of *Mycobacterium ulcerans*, the causative agent of Buruli ulcer. *Genome Res* 2007; 17: 192–200.

4. Wilson, M. D., Boakye, D. A., Mosi, L., Asiedu, K. In the case of transmission of *Mycobacterium ulcerans* in Buruli ulcer disease *Acanthamoeba* species stand accused. *Ghana Med J* 2011; 45: 1–4.

5. Eddyani, M., De Jonckheere, J. F., Durnez, L., Suykerbuyk, P., Leirs, H., *et al.* Occurrence of free-living amoebae in communities of low and high endemicity for Buruli ulcer in southern Benin. *Appl Environ Microbiol* 2008; 74: 6547–6553.

6. Ablordey, A., Kotlowski, R., Swings, J., Portaels, F. PCR amplification with primers based on IS2404 and GC-rich repeated sequence reveals polymorphism in *Mycobacterium ulcerans*. *J Clin Microbiol* 2005; 43 (1): 448-451.

7. Ablordey, A., Swings, J., Hubans, C., Chemlal, K., Locht, C., Portaels, F. Supply P. Multilocus variable-number tandem repeat typing of *Mycobacterium ulcerans*. *J Clin Microbiol.* 2005; 43(4): 1546-1551.

8. Ablordey, A., Hilty, M., Stragier, P., Swings, J., Portaels, F. Comparative nucleotide sequence analysis of polymorphic variable-number tandem-repeat loci in Mycobacterium ulcerans. J Clin Microbiol. 2005; 43 (10): 5281-5284.

9. Stragier, P., Ablordey, A., Meyers, W.M., Portaels, F. Genotyping Mycobacterium ulcerans and Mycobacterium marinum by using mycobacterial interspersed repetitive units. J Bacteriol 2005; 187(5):1639-1647.

10. Hilty, M., Yeboah-Manu, D., Boakye, D., Mensah-Quainoo, E., Rondini, S, et al. Genetic diversity in Mycobacterium ulcerans isolates from Ghana revealed by a newly identified locus containing a variable number of tandem repeats. J Bacteriol 2006; 188:1462–1465. doi:10.1128/JB.188.4.1462-1465.2006.

11. Stragier, P., Ablordey, A., Bayonne, L.M., Lugor, Y.L., Sindani, I.S., Suykerbuyk, P., Wabinga, H., Meyers, W.M., Portaels, F. Heterogeneity among Mycobacterium ulcerans isolates from Africa. Emerg Infect Dis 2006; 12(5): 844-847.

12. Ablordey, A., Fonteyne, P-A., Stragier, P., Vandamme, P., Portaels. F. Identification of a new VNTR locus in Mycobacterium ulcerans for potential strain discrimination among African isolates. Clin Microbiol Infec 2007; 13 (7): 734-736

13. Stragier, P., Ablordey, A., Durnez, L., Portaels, F. VNTR analysis differentiates Mycobacterium ulcerans and IS2404 positive mycobacteria. Syst Appl Microbiol 2007; 30: 525-530.

14. Röltgen, K., Qi W., Ruf, M-T., Mensah-Quainoo, E., Pidot, S.J., et al. Single nucleotide polymorphism typing of Mycobacterium ulcerans Reveals Focal Transmission of Buruli Ulcer in a Highly Endemic Region of Ghana. PLoS Negl Trop Dis 2010; 4:e751. doi:10.1371/journal.pntd.0000751.

15. Gryseels, S., Amissah, D., Durnez, L., Vandelannoote, K., Leirs, H., Jonckheere, J.D., Silva, M. T., Portaels, F., Ablordey, A., Eddyani M. Amoebae as potential environmental hosts for Mycobacterium ulcerans and other mycobacteria, but doubtful actors in Buruli ulcer Epidemiology. PLoS Negl Trop Dis 2012; 6(8):e1764. doi:10.1371/journal.pntd.0001764

16. Durnez, L., Stragier, P., Roebben, K., Ablordey, A., Leirs, H., et al. A comparison of DNA extraction procedures for the detection of Mycobacterium ulcerans, the causative agent of Buruli ulcer, in clinical and environmental specimens. J Microbiol Methods 2009 76:152–158.

17. Fyfe, J. A., Lavender, C. J., Johnson, P. D., Globan, M., Sievers, A., Azuolas, J., *et al*. Development and application of two multiplex real-time PCR assays for the detection of *Mycobacterium ulcerans* in clinical and environmental samples. *Appl Environ Microbiol* 2007; 73: 4733-4740.

18. Page, F. C. An illustrated key to freshwater and soil amoebae. Ambleside: UK: Freshwater Biological Association. 1976

19. De Jonckheere, J. F., Brown, S. The identification of vahlkampfiid amoebae by ITS sequencing. *Protist* 2005; 156: 89–96.

20. De Jonckheere, J. F. Sequence variation in the ribosomal internal transcribed spacers, including the 5.8S rDNA, of Naegleria spp. *Protist* 1998; 149: 221–228.

21. Schroeder, J. M., Booton, G. C., Hay, J., Niszl, I. A., Seal, D.V., *et al*. Use of subgenic 18S ribosomal DNA PCR and sequencing for genus and genotype identification of Acanthamoebae from humans with keratitis and from sewage sludge. *J Clin Microbiol* 2001; 39:1903–1911.

22. Johnson, P. D., Azuolas, J., Lavender, C. J. *et al*. *Mycobacterium ulcerans* in mosquitoes captured during outbreak of Buruli ulcer, southeastern Australia. *Emerg Infect Dis* 2007; 13:1653–1660

23. Williamson, H. R., Benbow, M. E., Nguyen, K. D., *et al*. Distribution of *Mycobacterium ulcerans* in Buruli ulcer endemic and non-endemic aquatic sites in Ghana. *PLoS Negl Trop Dis* 2008; 2:e205.

24. Lavender, C., Globan, M., Fyfe, J. A. M. *et al*.Buruli ulcer disease in travellers and differentiation of *Mycobacterium ulcerans* strains from northern Australia. *J Clin Microbiol* 2012; 50 (11): 3717-21.

# Chapter 12
## Improving Buruli Ulcer Diagnosis and Analysis of Delay in Wound Healing

*Dorothy Yeboah-Manu, Kobina Ampah, Samuel Aboagye,*
*Evelyn Owusu-Mireku, Grace Kpeli and Emelia Danso*

## Introduction

After tuberculosis and leprosy, Buruli ulcer (BU), which is caused by the environmental pathogen *Mycobacterium ulcerans*, is the most common mycobacterial infection in immuno-competent humans. Buruli ulcer affects impoverished populations living in wetlands, and areas where the environment has been greatly disturbed by such activities as deforestation and mining. The global burden of BU is not known, because of the lack of an efficient reporting system in most endemic countries.[1] However, it is now known that BU is endemic in at least 32 tropical countries of Africa, Western Pacific, Asia, the Indian Ocean and Latin America. Most cases are reported from West and Central African countries, where it occurs in remote areas, with limited access to health (Figure 12.1).[2] The worst affected region is within countries lying along the Gulf of Guinea in West Africa, where BU has replaced leprosy as the second most common mycobacterial disease, after tuberculosis. Cases have been detected in all the countries with Ghana, Côte d'Ivoire, Togo, Cameroon and Benin recording the highest number of cases.[2]

The first documented case of Buruli ulcer in Ghana was a patient from Amasaman at the Korle Bu Teaching Hospital in 1971.[3] A national case search performed in 1999 yielded a crude (national) BU prevalence rate of 20.7/100,000 and demonstrated that BU was the second most common mycobacteriosis in the country after tuberculosis.[3] In that study, diagnosis of both active and healed lesions was based solely on clinical grounds without any microbiological confirmation. A national BU control programme was therefore established and since then, 32 of the 166 districts across the nation continuously report BU. Through this passive surveillance system, over 11,000 cases were reported between 1993 and 2006 mainly from 6 of the 10 regions of Ghana.[4] The national programme still reports annually about 1,000 new cases from various health facilities in Ghana. Although BU affects all age groups in both sexes, it affects mainly children 15 years of age and below in Africa, with reported prevalence ranging between 45% and 70% in different areas.[4] Most of the lesions are located on the legs, feet, arms and hands.

*Mycobacterium ulcerans* is believed to have evolved from the water pathogen, *M. marinum,* by acquiring a giant plasmid of size 174kbp.[5] This plasmid harbours the synthetic machinery required for the production of the main virulent factor of the pathogen, the polyketide macrolide toxin called mycolactone. Mycolactone is cyto-toxic. It produces a necrotising effect in guinea pigs, which histologically, is found to be similar to that seen in human patients.[6] In addition it has *in vitro* activity against a number of immune cells, including those important for the control of mycobacterial infection such as neutrophils, macrophages and monocytes.[7]

After successful entry, the organism confines itself to the subcutaneous tissues and the overlaying skin, where it multiplies. The incubation period is variable, and has been approximated to range from 2 weeks to 3 years, with an average of 2 to 3 months.[8] After establishment of infection, secretion of the toxin by the microbe causes extensive necrotic damage to the host tissues, particularly the dermis, panniculus, and fascia and the suppression of immune response. Histological analysis of early lesions reveals extensive cutaneous tissue necrosis with large numbers of extracellular bacilli in clumps and scanty inflammatory cells, which may be the result of the immunosuppressive action of the toxin.[9] The early presentation of the disease varies between different people and geographical areas. The disease begins typically as a painless nodule under the skin at the site of the trauma. In some geographical areas, e.g. Australia, the first manifestation is a papule rather than the firm, painless nodule. In the more serious forms it is believed that due to the rapid spread of infection, the localized nodular-ulcerative stage starts as a plaque or oedematous plaque. After a few weeks, if left untreated, the nodule gradually enlarges and erodes through the skin surface, leaving a well-demarcated ulcer with a necrotic slough in the base and widely undermined edges.[5]

Currently the exact mode of transmission of M. ulcerans is still not clarified. However, BU affects people in scattered foci and endemic foci are usually associated with wetlands in hot and humid climates.[10] In this chapter we discuss how the NMIMR established diagnostic tools such as culture, PCR and monitored cases on treatment to understand causes of delay in wound healing. In addition it discusses some socioeconomic interventions put in place to improve early case detection and adherence to treatment.

# Improving and Establishment of Laboratory Confirmation Facility in Ghana

## Introduction

At the beginning of the global efforts to fight BU, there was no laboratory in endemic countries with the expertise and infrastructure to microbiologically confirm BU, either by culture, PCR or histopathology. Cases were defined only on clinical grounds or transported abroad for confirmation.[11] The presentation of typical indolent, painless, undermined edges and necrotic slough lesion allows a straightforward diagnosis of ulcerative lesions. However, diagnosis is more difficult, for the nodule, plaque, oedema and atypical forms, which may be confused with other skin diseases.[7] Thus, reconfirmation of clinically diagnosed cases is very important to prevent unnecessary surgical excision and/ or antimycobacterial drug treatment of patients with non-BU lesions, and for epidemiological surveillance. Mycobacterium ulcerans isolation from clinical samples is a difficult process due to factors such as its slow growth and contamination of cultures by other faster growing bacteria. The recorded sensitivity is very low, and as low as 13% has been recorded.[12] At the same time, M. ulcerans isolates are needed for understanding disease micro-epidemiology, surveillance of drug resistance and monitoring response to therapy.

# Approach

## Pathological samples

Samples that were used for the analysis include tissue biopsy, swab and fine needle aspirate (FNA). These specimens were collected from patients that were diagnosed clinically as BU. While swab specimens were taken from the undermined edges of ulcerative lesions, FNA was taken from the centre (weakest point) on non-ulcerative lesions, while biopsy was taken during surgery from both types. Samples were collected either through passive case recruitment that were presenting at health facilities and or during active case search in communities. Swab samples that are received in our laboratory from outside the Greater Accra Region, usually come as dry swabs and have spent between 2 days and 1 month in transit. To optimize bacteria release from the swab sample, two procedures were evaluated using 20 paired samples. In the first process, swab specimen(s) from the same lesion were pooled together and soaked in sterile PBS for 30 minutes, which was followed by vortexing for 2 minutes. In the second process, swab specimen(s) from the same lesion were pooled together and soaked for 30 minutes in a tube containing sterile PBS and ten 3-mm-diameter undrilled glass beads (Merck, Darmstadt, Germany). The specimen was then vortexed for 2 minutes. The effectiveness of the two procedures was evaluated semi-quantitatively by microscopy and real-time PCR. Thereafter, the better of the two procedures was used for subsequent sample processing. In addition, blood samples were collected from BU cases and contacts for the preparation of sera, which were used in evaluation of sero-diagnosis as rapid and easier methods for diagnosis of BU.

## *Optimisation of cultivation of* M. ulcerans

Care was taken not to contaminate all collected samples and they were stored at 4°C in modified Dubos transport medium supplemented with 10% oleic acid albumin-dextrose-catalase (KC Biologicals, Lenexa, Kans. USA), 2% PANTA Plus (Becton Dickinson, Franklin Lakes, N.Y. USA), and 0.5% agar (Difco). In most of the cases, samples were transported and processed in the laboratory within seven days. Tissue samples were cut into smaller pieces, homogenized, and suspended in 8ml of Dulbecco's phosphate-buffered saline.(PH .74) While swab samples from the same lesion were vortexed for 2 minutes in 50 ml tubes containing glass beads (3 mm diameter) to disperse off as much as possible all bacteria attached to the swab into the PBS. The obtained suspension was divided into equal aliquots of 2ml each. Aliquots were then used for evaluation of the different decontamination procedures.[13] After decontamination the homogenates were concentrated by centrifugation, and were inoculated in duplicates on different solid media for evaluation.

## Optimisation of microscopy

The bacteria suspensions obtained as already described for the different pathological samples were concentrated by centrifuging at 3,000 × g for 15 minutes. After decanting the supernatant, the sediment was used for smear preparation, fixed and stained using the Ziehl-Neelsen procedure. Slides were graded using the International Union Against Tuberculosis and Lung Disease (IUATLD) scale. One-tenth of all the slides were blindly evaluated by an independent technician. A discordant reading was resolved by a second assessor.

## Setting-up of the polymerase chain reaction (PCR) Analysis Centre

This was done in response to a call from the Ghana Health Service requesting the NMIMR to help confirm laboratory-diagnosed BU cases. We optimised DNA extraction using the commercial kit from QIAGEN, Hillden, Germany, using the manufacturer's instruction with slight modification. The polymerase chain reaction (PCR) primers and reaction condition that was established was as reported earlier.[14]

# Results and Discussion

## Cultivation optimisation

In previously reported studies,[15] clinical specimens were collected in remote endemic areas of Africa and shipped to research or diagnostic laboratories in Europe or North America. A major contribution of the success of our work was the establishment of a very successful culturing system in an endemic country. As indicated in Table 12. 1, our culture optimisation achieved a recovery rate of about 70% when isolating from tissue biopsies obtained from surgery, 50% from swabs and 41.2% from FNA specimens. We believe the reduction in isolation rate was due to the smaller amount of material collected by the last two pathological samples. Our finding for the first time indicated that positive cultures can be obtained from FNA. With the introduction of antibiotic treatment and an increase in early case detection programmes we envisage FNA will be the main sample for laboratory analysis. This finding is good as we need isolates for micro-epidemiological studies as well as drug-resistance surveillance.

*Mycobacterium sp* differ in their preference for carbon source utilisation, with variation across the genus. This is particularly true with regard to glycerol utilisation. Under laboratory conditions glycerol is the preferred carbon source for a number of mycobacterial species, including M. *tuberculosis*. However, M. *bovis*, M. *africanum* and M. *microtti* are all unable to use glycerol as a sole carbon source, and pyruvate is therefore routinely added to glycerinated media to enable growth.[16] The preferred carbon source for M. *ulcerans* had not been established. Our study showed for the first time that M. *ulcerans* prefers glycerol to pyruvate as a source of carbon and so a medium for M. *ulcerans* should contain glycerol. The number of positive cultures was greatly reduced when a medium containing pyruvate was used for isolation; our findings also indicated that M. *ulcerans* grows better in LJ medium when compared to Ogawa medium. Finally, when we compared the standard oxalic acid decontamination which includes both 5% oxalic acid and sodium hydroxide to a simplified procedure that involves only 5% oxalic acid, we found that the standard decontamination procedure was harsher than our simplified method (Table 12.1). In addition to culture being the most definite method for microbiological confirmation of clinical diagnosis, which has been used for monitoring treatment, we have raised a large collection of isolates that is helpful in the understanding of the epidemiology of the microbe being studied. This is crucial in the case of M. *ulcerans* for which current knowledge is very scanty.

Table 12.1:  Performance of different conditions that was evaluated to improve primary *M. ulcerans* isolation

| Criteria | Number of samples analysed, N | Number positive n (%) | P value |
|---|---|---|---|
| Specimen Type | | | |
| Swab | 20 | 10 (50) | 0.752 |
| Tissue | 164 | 112 (68.3) | 0.000 |
| FNA | 12 | 5 (41.7) | 0.683 |
| Media | | | |
| Lowenstein Jenseen | 164 | 112 (68.3) | 0.000 |
| Ogawa | 164 | 88 (53.6) | 0.224 |
| Carbon Source | | | |
| Glycerol | 164 | 112 (68.3) | 0.000 |
| Pyruvate | 164 | 78 (47.6) | 0.439 |
| Decontamination | | | |
| Standard Oxalic Acid | 20 | 1 (5) | 0.000 |
| In-house simplified oxalic acid | 20 | 10 (50) | 0.752 |

## Optimisation of microscopy

While PCR is rapid and sensitive, it is out of the reach of the peripheral centres where BU is prevalent, but all these centres have capacity to conduct ZN microscopy. Swabs soaked in PBS were vortexed with or without glass beads. Suspensions were subsequently evaluated by microscopy after ZN staining and semi-quantitative IS2404 real-time (RT) PCR. Included in the comparative study were 19 BU lesions testing positive by RT-PCR (cycle threshold [Ct] ≤ 39) after sample processing with glass beads. The addition of glass beads increased the microscopic detection of AFBs from 21% (4/19) to 58% (11/19). Six out of 19 (32%) lesions that were negative by RT-PCR vortexed without glass beads became positive when glass beads were used. To increase the sensitivity of microscopy, we further concentrated supernatants by centrifugation. When we compared this optimised microscopy procedure to IS2404 PCR as the gold-standard diagnostic method, the sensitivity and specificity of microscopy were 57.1%

(44/77) and 95.7% (22/23), respectively. Further analysis indicated that the sensitivity can be improved when more than one sample is analysed. We recommend that microscopic confirmation of BU at peripheral centres should be encouraged, as is being done for TB, and that a percentage of samples could be sent to reference laboratory for quality control. In addition, we do agree that for the confirmation of a new endemic focus, the use of PCR should be encouraged.

## Establishment of a National BU Diagnostic Centre

With the introduction of antibiotic treatment of Buruli ulcer by daily oral rifampicin and streptomycin injections for eight weeks (SR8) as first-line anti-BU treatment strategy, laboratory confirmation became very necessary to avoid unnecessary drug treatment as a result of false clinical diagnosis. However, the infrastructure and expertise for the gold-standard method for laboratory confirmation, which is PCR detection of the insertion sequence IS2404, is unavailable within the health facilities in endemic African countries, including facilities of the Ghana Health Service. The NMIMR responded to this by setting up a laboratory for confirming cases by PCR (Figure12.1) and also for quality controlling clinical diagnosis.[17] Between 2007 and 2011, we have analysed by PCR, 1,392 samples from seven regions of Ghana; The only regions that we have not yet received samples from are Western, Upper East and Upper West. The average positivity rate was 62.3%, with the range from 56.1% to 80%. Majority of the samples (71.4%) were received from the Greater-Accra Region followed by the Eastern Region (13.3%).

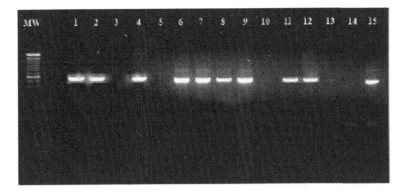

*Figure 12.1: Gel electrograph of PCR products of patients with lesions suspected to be Buruli ulcer. Lane MW is 100kb ladder, 3, and 10 are swabs from patients with ulcers not caused by M. ulcerans; lanes 13, 14 and 15 are extraction, negative and positive controls while the remaining lanes are swabs from Buruli ulcer patients.*

# Treatment of Buruli ulcer disease – Analysis of delay in wound healing

## Introduction

Buruli ulcer (BU) has traditionally been considered a disease that can only be cured with surgery. This belief developed because of the massively destructive nature of the disease, early reports which suggested that wide surgical excision was the only effective treatment[18] and in the antibiotic era, early trials with clofazimine[19] and rifampicin/clofazimine[20] which demonstrated only marginal benefits. Recently, WHO has introduced new provisional antibiotic treatment guidelines for BU following a successful pilot study conducted in Ghana which confirmed that human lesions could be sterilised with antibiotics.[21] This was supported by encouraging reports of success with this protocol in a case series from Benin.[22] BU is treated first by daily injections of streptomycin and oral rifampicin for eight weeks (SR8) and surgery only to correct deformities and in few instances to improve wound healing. This has reduced the rate of recurrence and centralised treatment. The protocol has led to a new approach to treatment with the potential to reduce cost, to allow delivery of care closer to the homes of patients, and to encourage patients to present earlier as the fear of major surgery is lessened. A prospective cohort study was therefore designed to confirm these excellent results, to build confidence in this new treatment strategy at the local level and to investigate the reason(s) why treatment may occasionally fail.

## Approach

### Study participants

Participants included in this study satisfied the WHO clinical definition for the different BU lesions that were microbiologically confirmed by at least *IS2404* PCR. Lesions were then categorized into;

(i) category I, which consisted of a lesion size of <5 cm at the widest diameter;

(ii) category II, which consisted of a lesion size of between 5cm and 15 cm at the widest diameter; and

(iii) category III, which consisted of a lesion size >15 cm at the widest diameter.

In addition patients were classified either as ulcerative, oedema, nodule and papule as well as having either single or multiple lesions.

Written informed consent was sought either from literate patients and verbally from patients who could not read before inclusion in the study. In the case of minors, consent was sought from their parents/ guardians. Ethical clearance for this study was obtained from the Institutional Review Board of the Noguchi Memorial Institute for Medical Research.

### BU case management and treatment monitoring

Wound dressing was immediately commenced upon clinical diagnosis and antibiotic treatment was initiated upon microbiological confirmation. Each patient was weighed and antibiotic (oral rifampicin at 10 mg/kg daily and intramuscular streptomycin at 15 mg/kg) was given daily for eight weeks. The directly observed treatment strategy was used to record case compliance of treatment using the WHO patient treatment cards (BU03) and compliance was recorded by ticking daily after taking the regimen. Wounds were assessed bi-weekly until healed; deteriorated wounds were further investigated for viability of *M. ulcerans*, secondary infection and in some of the cases, additional co-founding illness such as HIV/AIDS and diabetes.

## Definitions

(i) **Successful treatment**: Treatment was considered "successful" when the lesions were completely healed (scarred without residual inflammation) upon completion of the eight-week antibiotic treatment or during the 24 weeks after starting treatment without adjunctive surgical excision.

(ii) **Loss to follow-up:** Patients were considered as "lost to follow-up" (defaulters) when they abandoned or refused treatment.

(iii) **Failed treatment:** Treatment was considered to have "failed" in the event of death related to *M. ulcerans* disease and/or the persistence of non-scarring lesions despite appropriate medical treatment after SR8 treatment.

(iv) **Improved treatment:** Participants whose wound looked clean, the lesion had reduced by 50% or more after SR8 treatment

## Results and Discussions

### Participants and history

The total number of suspected cases recruited was 475, out of which, 357 (75%) comprising 183 females and 174 males were confirmed microbiologically as BU. The arithmetic mean age of the confirmed cases was 30. median 28, mode 10 years. However, unlike previous reports that indicated that around 70% of cases are children aged 15 years and below, we found only 111 of the 350 (31.7%) of BU cases in general were in this age bracket. Three hundred and nineteen (89.36%) of these presented with single lesions, 35 (9.8%) presented with multiple lesions and 3 (0.84%) did not indicate the number of lesions. Ninety-one (25.49%) of them presented with Category I lesions while 93 (26.05%) and 167 (46.78%) presented with Categories II and III respectively; 6 (1.68%) of them were not indicated. This indicates that most of the cases reported late and therefore points to the need to intensify education and early detection activities.

## Treatment and outcome

Two hundred and eighty-six patients received streptomycin and rifampicin combined antibiotic treatment and of these, 197 (68.9%) had a successful outcome; 20 (7.0%) patients had their lesions improved; 25 (8.7%) patients were lost to follow-up and 44 patients (15.4%) failed treatment. Thus, all together 75.9% patients had a positive outcome. One hundred and thirty-seven (69.5%) of the treatment success cases healed without any surgical intervention and the duration of treatment for this group was between 8 and 24 weeks (median duration of 12 weeks) while that of the failed cases was between 26 and 96 weeks (median duration of 36 weeks).This finding is comparable to other studies that indicate that most cases that reported early heal early and treatment can be done without surgery.[17] As a result of this finding as it will be discussed in the next chapter, the NMIMR is piloting an early case detection intervention in the Ga-South District. Further laboratory investigation revealed that factors that influence treatment failure were: secondary infection (Figure 12.2), prolonged viability of M. ulcerans (Figure 12.3), health-seeking behaviour and co-morbidities.

## 1.   Secondary infection and healing delay

Thirty-one out of 86 BU lesions with clinical signs of bacterial super-infection after completion of SR8 treatment were sampled for laboratory investigation. The clinical signs of cases indicative of secondary infection included: localised pain, localised heat, cellulitis, viscous/purulent discharge and oedema, discolouration of tissues both within and at the wound margins and offensive odour. The time in which infection was detected ranged from 4 weeks to 15 months after completion of SR8. Seven (22.6%%) of the 31 lesions were not confirmed by aerobic bacterial count analysis to be infected, as the total plate count ranged only between $1.3 \times 10^3$ and $8.9 \times 10^5$ CFU/ml (average $2.7 \times 10^5$ CFU/ml). The remaining 24 (77.4%) lesions that were microbiologically confirmed as infected had plate counts ranging between 1.2 x $10^6$ and 3.5 x $10^9$ CFU/ml (average value of 1.2 x$10^9$). *P. aeruginosa* (n=8; 32%), *P. mirabilis* (n=5; 20%) and *S. aureus* (n=3; 12%) dominated among the isolates. Tissue samples from 20 out of 31 of the microbiologically analyzed lesions showing clinical signs of secondary infection after completion of SR8 were also analyzed by histopathology, since the responsible clinicians decided to perform a wound debridement. Microbiological analysis had categorized 16 of the lesions as infected and four as contaminated. None of the microbiologically contaminated wounds presented in the histopathological analysis with a detectable secondary infection. In contrast 12/16 (75%) of the lesions classified microbiologically as infected presented with a secondary infection either with cocci, rods or both. Secondary infection was mainly observed in the stratum corneum (6/12; 50%) or on the open ulcer surface (3/12; 25%) and also (3/12; 25%) in deeper inside the excised tissue.

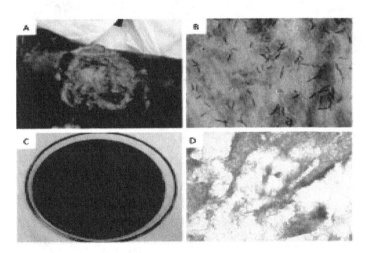

*Figure 12.2: A: Clinical presentation of Buruli ulcer patient with an infected wound 13 weeks after streptomycin/rifampicin treatment. B: Direct smear examination after Gram staining showing large numbers of pus cells. C: Primary culture on blood agar and D: Histological sections after staining with methylene blue indicating clumps of rods.*

## 2. Prolonged viability of *M. ulcerans* cells

Twenty cases with delayed wound healing after SR8 were sampled after antibiotic treatment for mycobacterial culture. Of these, 12 (60%) received SR12. Eight of them (40%) were culture positive after antibiotic treatment. However, preliminary analysis does not indicate that these isolates were resistant to any of the two antibiotics used for treatment. Most of the cases within this category presented with large ulcers; probably the delay in clearing the pathogen may be due to poor blood flow as a result of massive dead tissue preventing the antibiotic from reaching site of infection. Such cases were healed through large excision and skin grafting.

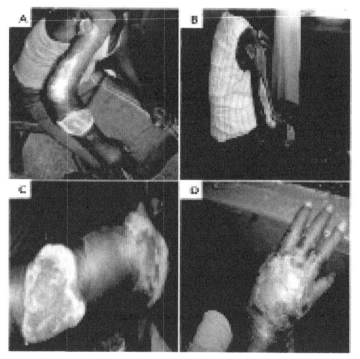

*Figure 12.3: Clinical presentation of a BU patient with four lesions that were all confirmed by at least IS2404 PCR. A: At first presentation, B: four weeks of SR8 treatment C/D: 8 Weeks after SR8, two of the lesions that did not improve were culture positive, indicating the presence of viable M. ulcerans cells.*

## 3.  Health-seeking behaviour

Health-seeking delay (p<0.019) and category of lesion seen (p<0.005) was found to be critical in determining the length of BU treatment (Table 12.2). As indicated by participants' lesion presentations and categories, a significant number of cases reported at the late stages, especially those that self-reported and were not found by active case search. Half (50%) of the 200 cases seen at the Amasaman District Hospital (ADH) sought help after six months with some (5%) reporting well over 10 years with very advanced lesions. Most cases (63%) received some form of traditional herbal preparations before coming to hospitals.

**Table 12.2:  The category of Buruli ulcer lesion presented at the health facility and duration of treatment**

| Lesion Category at Presentation | Time Range from Start of Treatment to Wound Healing (weeks) | Median Time from Start of Treatment to Wound Healing (weeks) |
|---|---|---|
| Category I | 8-12 | 8 |
| Category II | 8-48 | 12 |
| Category III | 12-96 | 24 |

## 4.  Co-infection with HIV/AIDS and other causes

After counselling, 50 cases were tested for HIV, and of these 12 (24%) were HIV positive, two of whom died during treatment, with some of them having severe secondary infection as well. In addition, six patients died due to severe anaemia as a result of their lesions becoming cancerous.

## Concluding Remarks

SR8 treatment is effective in treating BU cases, and those who presented with Category 1 lesions are usually healed within three months with no surgical intervention. However, a reasonable number of cases still have to stay for extended periods of time (even more than two years) in hospital after completion of antibiotic treatment. Our findings indicate that, depending on the type of lesion and individual factors, different mechanisms contribute to retarded wound healing. These include:

- Secondary infection of wounds;
- Prolonged surviving *M. ulcerans* cells;
- HIV/AIDS co-infection;
- Late case reporting at hospitals and clinics, resulting in the presentation of large ulcers.

## Acknowledgment

We are grateful to the productive collaboration I have had with Prof. Gerd Pluschke, Swiss Tropical and Public Health Institute. We wish to thank all the health facilities we received samples from especially the Amasaman District Hospital and the Obom Health Centre, and the National Buruli Ulcer Control Programme. We also appreciate the study participants, their parents and guardians and USS Options Foundation for financial support

## Reference

1. World Heatlh Organisation. WHO Global Buruli Ulcer Initiative (GBUI). Available at: http://www.who.int/gtb-buruli.

2. Porten, K., Sailor, K., Comte, E., Njikap, A., Sobry, A. *et al.* Prevalence of Buruli ulcer in Akonolinga Health District, Cameroon: results of a cross sectional survey. (2009). *PLoS Negl Trop Dis* 3(6): e466. doi:10.1371/journal.pntd.0000466

3. Ackumey, M. M., Kwakye-Maclean, C., Ampadu, E. O., de Savigny, D., Weiss, M. G. *et al.* Health services for Buruli ulcer control: lessons from a field study in Ghana. (2011). *PLoS Negl Trop Dis* 5(6): e1187. doi:10.1371/journal.pntd.0001187

4. Amofah, G., Bonsu, F., Tetteh, C., Okrah, J., Asamoah, K. *et al.* Buruli ulcer in Ghana: results of a national case search. (2002). *Emerg InfectDis* 8(2): 167-170

5. Stinear, T. P., Mve-Obiang, A., Small, P .L., Frigui, W., Pryor, M.J. *et al.* Giant plasmid-encoded polyketide synthases produce the macrolide toxin of *Mycobacterium ulcerans*. (2004). *Proc Natl Acad Sci USA* 101(5): 1345-9.

6.  George, K. M., Pascopella, L., Welty, D. M. and Small, P. L. C. A *Mycobacterium ulcerans* toxin, mycolactone, causes apoptosis in Guinea pig ulcers and tissue culture cells. (2000). *Infect Imm* 68(2): 877-883.

7.  Asiedu, K., Scherpbier, R. and Raviglione, M. Buruli ulcer: press release WHO/2000. Geneva: World Health Organization.

8.  Hong, H., Demangel, C., Pidot, S. J., Leadlay, P. F. and Stinear, T. Mycolactones: immunosuppressive and cytotoxic polyketides produced by aquatic mycobacterial. (2008). *Nat Prod Rep* 25(3): 447–454. doi:10.1039/b803101k

9.  Abalos, F. M., Aguiar, J., Guedenon, S. R. A., Portaels, F. and Meyers W.M. *Mycobacterium ulcerans* infection (Buruli ulcer): a case report of the disseminated non ulcerative form. (2000). *Ann Diagn Pathol* 4: 386-390.

10. Pszolla, N., Sarkar, M. R, Strecker, W., Kern, P., Kinzl, L. *et al*. Buruli ulcer: a systemic disease. (2003). *Clin Infect Dis* 37: e78-e82

11. van der Werf, T.S., van der Graaf, W.T., Tappero, J.W. and Asiedu, K. *Mycobacterium ulcerans* infection. (1999). *Lancet* 354:1013-1018.

12. Yeboah-Manu, D., Danso, E., Ampah, K., Asante-Poku, A., Nakobu, Z. *et al*. Isolation of *Mycobacterium ulcerans* from swab and fine-needle-aspiration specimens. (2011). *J Clin Microbiol* 49(5): 1997–1999. doi:10.1128/JCM.02279-10

13. Yeboah-Manu, D., Bodmer, T., Mensah-Quainoo, E., Owusu, S., Ofori-Adjei, D. *et al*. Evaluation of decontamination methods and growth media for primary isolation of *Mycobacterium ulcerans* from surgical specimens. (2004). *J Clin Microbiol* 42(12): 5875- 5876.doi:10.1128/JCM.42.12.5875-5876.2004

14. Guimaraes-Peres, A., Portaels, F., de Rijk, P., Fissette, K., Pattyn, S.R. *et al*. Comparison of two PCRs for detection of *Mycobacterium ulcerans*. (1999). *J Clin Microbiol* 37(1): 206–208.

15. Siegmund, V., Adjei, O., Nitschke, J., Thompson, W., Klutse, E. *et al*. Dry reagent–based polymerase chain reaction compared with other laboratory methods available for the diagnosis of Buruli ulcer disease. (2007). *Clin Infect Dis* 45(1):68-75.doi:10.1086/518604

16. Keating, L. A.,Wheeler, P. R.,Mansoor, H.,Inwald, J. K.,Dale, J. *et al*. The pyruvate requirement of some members of the *Mycobacterium tuberculosis* complex is due to an inactive pyruvate kinase: implications for *in vivo* growth. (2005). *Mol Microbiol* 56(1):163-74.

17. Mensah-Quainoo, E., Yeboah-Manu, D., Asebi, C., Patafuor F,Ofori-Adjei, D. *et al*. Diagnosis of *Mycobacterium ulcerans* infection (Buruli ulcer) at a treatment centre in Ghana: a retrospective analysis of

laboratory results of clinically diagnosed cases. (2008). *Trop Med Int Health*13(2): 191–198.

18. Revill, W. D., Morrow, R. H., Pike, M. C., and Ateng, J. A controlled trial of the treatment of *Mycobacterium ulcerans* infection with clofazimine. (1973). *Lancet* 2: 873–877.

19. Espey, D. K., Djomand, G., Diomande, I., Dosso, M., Saki, M.Z. *et al.* A pilot study of treatment of Buruli ulcer with rifampin and dapsone. (2002). *Int J Infect Dis* 6: 60–65.

20. Etuaful, S., Carbonnelle, B., Grosset, J., Lucas, S., Horsfield, C. *et al.* Efficacy of the combination rifampin-streptomycin in preventing growth of *Mycobacterium ulcerans* in early lesions of Buruli ulcer in humans. (2005). *Antimicrob Agents Chemother* 49: 3182–3186.

21. Chauty, A., Ardant, M. F., Adeye, A., Euverte, H., Guedenon, A. *et al.* Promising clinical efficacy of streptomycin-rifampin combination for treatment of Buruli ulcer (*Mycobacterium ulcerans* disease). (2007). *Antimicrob Agents Chemother* 51: 4029–4035.

22. Barogui, Y., Johnson, R. C., van der Werf, T. S., Sopoh, G., Dossou, A. *et al.* Functional limitations after surgical or antibiotic treatment for Buruli ulcer in Benin. (2009). *Am J Trop Med Hyg* 81(1): 82-87.

# Chapter 13
## Social Interventions for Buruli Ulcer Control in Obom Sub-District of Ghana

*Collins K Ahorlu, Eric Koka and Dorothy Yeboah-Manu*

## Background

Buruli ulcer (BU) is generally referred to as a re-emerging disease particularly in West Africa, where the prevalence in some cases could be higher than tuberculosis. Children aged 15 years and below are the worst affected in this endemic region.[1,2] The disease begins typically as a painless nodule under the skin however, in some areas a papule rather than firm and painless nodule is the first manifestation. If not treated early, it gradually enlarges and erodes through the skin surface, leaving a well-demarcated ulcer with a necrotic slough in the base and widely undermined edges, which is the hallmark of the disease. Although, fatality among BU sufferers is low, they suffer a great deal of morbidity and prolonged treatment delay could lead to bone involvement, functional disabilities such as amputation of limbs and other vital organs. These notwithstanding, many cases reach biomedical treatment centres late due to various reasons.[3,4] In Ghana, about 1000 cases are reported yearly, giving a nationwide prevalence of 20.7/100,000 in 1998. However, the district-level prevalence of the Ga South District, where this study took place was 87.7/100,000 population.[2,5]

Buruli Ulcer (BU) is caused by the environmental pathogen *Mycobacterium ulcerans* but its mode of transmission is still not known. While we wait for a better understanding of BU transmission dynamics, it is essential to implement interventions that enhance access to early effective treatment. Such efforts will require community mobilization and involvement in making use of available BU control tools in more innovative ways to promote early case detection, diagnosis and treatment.

Most social science studies on Buruli ulcer have discussed various socio-cultural aspects of the disease and tends to focus on BU-related beliefs, perceptions and the economic cost of the disease and how these factors affect early case detection and treatment-seeking behaviour negatively.[6-13] Most of these studies concluded that Information, Education and Communication (IEC) interventions were needed to empower affected families to take appropriate actions related to treatment seeking.[14] However, it has been argued that "all over the world those who do not comply are those least able to comply"[15] Social science research therefore needs to go beyond the description of existing problems and putting forward health education as the magic bullet that will improve treatment seeking for BU. This chapter departs from this position to focus on how to intervene at the level of both the affected persons and the care providers in order to remove existing barriers to early diagnosis and treatment bearing in mind that the challenge is not availability of treatment but inability to access the existing treatment by those who need it most.

In the past, BU was treated mainly by surgical intervention, necessitating centralised management of cases at bigger health facilities. However, since 2006, the WHO-recommended first-line treatment for BU is oral rifampicin (10 mg/kg) plus intramuscular streptomycin injection (15 mg/kg), both given daily for eight weeks under supervision.[16] Although daily injections for eight weeks is not a pleasant experience to go through, it has proven to be very effective in curing BU patients, especially when accessed at the early stage of the disease. This chapter focuses on interventions that were implemented to encourage patients to complete treatment, no matter how unpleasant it might have been. Findings were discussed in line with access to a health care framework,[17] from the viewpoint of availability, accessibility, affordability, adequacy and acceptability of the services that clients are expected to receive from a facility.

# Approach

## Study area

The study was conducted in the Obom sub-district, Ga South Municipality with an estimated population of 210,727. BU is highly endemic in Ga South Municipality, which is one of the municipalities in Ghana that continue to report a large proportion of the severe forms of ulcerative BU cases. The Obom health centre is the second largest health facility in the municipality besides the district hospital at Weija.

## Study design

This was a descriptive qualitative study designed to compare pre- and post-intervention data from community perspectives. The design helped to determine the effectiveness of selected social interventions for early case identification, diagnosis and treatment at the health care facility to reduce treatment dropout and default. Also, facility records of patients were reviewed to generate data on treatment default and dropout rates among those who went to the clinic six months prior to the commencement of the interventions. Informed consent was obtained from all respondents and caretakers of patients under 18 years of age. The project received approval from the Noguchi Memorial Institute's Institutional Review Board.

## Interventions

Two sets of related interventions were implemented in two phases. The first intervention phase was from July to December 2010 and comprised of community outreach education and screening, re-training of community-based volunteers who were given bicycles and provided with transportation to convey patients to and from the clinic for daily treatment. The second intervention was from January to June 2011 and comprised all the interventions implemented at the first phase in addition to formation of a former BU patients' club, training and collaboration with traditional healers and provision of breakfast to patients after treatment at the clinic.

All the various interventions were implemented with the aim of improving early case detection/diagnosis, treatment/management, ensuring treatment completion through enhanced community involvement and support, and increasing access to health care services for BU patients. Interventions also aimed at supporting the health care system (clinics) to respond promptly and appropriately through early laboratory testing and treatment support. Community consent was sought from chiefs and elders of all participating communities to perform case search, early recognition, diagnosis and treatment in the communities.

### Community outreach to enhance early case detection and treatment:

This intervention involved showing of BU-related documentary films and pictures of people who had successfully completed biomedical treatments and were healed. All the pictures used were of people who had given consent to the research team to use their pictures for educational purposes. This activity was done during the early hours of the evening (between 7 and 9 pm). The documentary film was interspersed with questions and answers. Screening for suspected BU cases was done the following morning by a team from Noguchi Memorial Institute for Medical Research supported by the environmental health officer in the sub-district and community assistants. Samples collected from suspected cases were sent to Noguchi Memorial Institute for Medical Research for laboratory confirmation.

### Re-training of community-based volunteers in BU case detection and referral:

Community-based volunteers were selected and trained by the Ghana Health Service to support health care delivery including BU. However, most of them were not active in the communities. Sixteen (16) of those within the study area were re-trained to actively search for suspected BU cases for referral to the clinic. To boost their morale, new bicycles were given to 12 of them who did not possess any. After the first six months of the interventions, evaluation reports showed that they were not doing much, so an amount of GH¢10 ($7) was paid to them for every case referred to the clinic and confirmed to be BU during the second phase of implementation. However, when a referred case is not confirmed as BU by the laboratory, then only the transportation cost for bringing the suspected patient to the clinic was covered. This was done so that no one would abuse the system for monetary gain.

### Formation of former BU patients clubs:

In order to encourage former patients to serve as treatment ambassadors, three former patients clubs were formed to promote early case finding and referral to the clinic for diagnosis and treatment. An amount of GH¢10 ($7) was paid to them for every case referred to the clinic that was confirmed as BU. Membership in the club was voluntary but one must have had BU and had been treated at the clinic.

### Provision of transportation to convey BU cases to and from the clinic:

Buruli ulcer is endemic in areas where transportation is limited and expensive and this was contributing to treatment default and dropout, and reduced school attendance, especially among affected school pupils. Transportation was therefore provided to convey cases to and from the clinic on a daily basis.

### Provision of breakfast to BU patients after drug administration:

One reason given by patients for defaulting and dropping out of treatment was that they felt hungry after taking the medications and in most cases had nothing to eat. So an arrangement was made to provide breakfast to them within a clinically acceptable time after taking the medications to see how this would affect clinic attendance and adherence to treatment. The breakfast cost GH¢1.00 ($0.70) per person/day.

### Training and collaboration with traditional healers:

At baseline, some traditional healers said they were willing to collaborate with the health system, so 10 of them were trained in BU case detection and referral. This was done in a manner that ensured mutual trust and respect. An amount of GH¢10 ($7) was paid to them for every case referred to the clinic that was confirmed as BU.

## Data collection

### Baseline and evaluation data collection

In-depth interview: Respondents for the qualitative data were BU patients (6), former patients (4), caretakers of BU patients (6), community volunteers (6), traditional healers (4) and clinic staff (2). The in-depth interview guide was designed to solicit information on general attitude to BU, expectations about biomedical treatments, early case detection, referrals, diagnosis, treatment and the challenges facing these processes. In all, 28 in-depth interviews were conducted at baseline, first evaluation and second evaluation. With the exception of the traditional healers, respondents were selected equitably from both genders. Respondents were randomly selected from a list prepared for each category of respondents, except for health workers, who were selected to represent those who take care of BU patients at the clinic. The in-depth interview guide was pre-tested and the results were used to refine the tool before the main data collection. The guide helped the interviewer to stay on course and manage deviations effectively. Two research assistants together with the first author conducted the interviews. At all the sessions, one person acted as a note taker and with permission from respondents, the interviews were tape-recorded.

### Clinic records review:

It was important to review patients' records at the clinic both at baseline and evaluation to demonstrate any changes that might have occurred as a result of interventions implemented. Baseline review was done from January–June 2010. This period was chosen because the clinic had fairly good records available. The first evaluation was done from July–December 2010 to coincide with the first phase of implementation while the second evaluation was done from January–June 2011 to correspond to the second phase of implementation. All treatment cards of BU patients were examined to record treatment start date, defaulting date, dropout date and completion date for each patient.

## Data analysis

Qualitative data were analysed using MAXQDA software for textual analysis. Variables of interest in the database were imported into MAXQDA as selection variables, which allowed the performance of phenomenological analysis on relevant coded segments from respondents for presentation. Representative narratives were presented to show the position of respondents on topics of interest before and after evaluation. The review data were analysed descriptively using EpiInfo (version 3.3.2) software.

## Results and Discussion

After 12 months' implementation, treatment default and dropout had reduced significantly from 58.8% and 52.9% at baseline to 1.5% and 1.5% respectively, a reduction of over 95%. The number of cases detected early went up significantly from 10 at baseline to 51 in 12 months, an increase of over 500%. There was a major increase in the number of patients referred by community-based volunteers, from four at baseline to 25 in 12 months, an increase of over 600%. All these could be attributed to the social interventions implemented, where cases were actively searched for and all suspected cases found referred to the clinic.

Table 13.1: Referral of patients to the clinic

| Variables | January-June 2010 (Before intervention) N = 16 (%) | July-December 2010 (Partial intervention) N= 39 (%) | January-June 2011 (Full intervention) N= 78 (%) |
|---|---|---|---|
| Community outreach | 2 (12.5) | 28 (71.7) | 30 (38.5) |
| Community volunteers | 4 (25.8) | 4 (10.3) | 25 (32.1) |
| Former patient | 0 | 1 (2.6) | 7 (8.9) |
| Self/relative | 10 (58.8) | 5 (12.8) | 14 (17.9) |
| Traditional healer | 0 | 1 (2.6) | 2 (2.6) |

The situation at baseline and evaluation were aptly demonstrated in the following narratives from care providers: *The problem of BU is that patients do not want to come for treatment*

*....I do not know whether it is because of the injection (daily for 56 days)..., you would have to see the wounds of those who came for treatment... very big and offensive, and difficult to manage...They have applied all sorts of materials on the wound before coming...sometimes, you don't know what to do than to transfer them to Amasaman for admission...* (clinic staff, IDI at baseline).

*As people who take care of these patients when they come to the clinic, especially dressing their wounds, I can say that the current intervention is very good... Now, more people are coming with very small wounds which are very easy to manage and we are all happy... It is our prayer that this will continue so that very soon there will be no BU in this area (clinic staff, IDI at evaluation).*

The social interventions implemented brought a lot of relief to the patients and the affected families in general. They were very happy and highly appreciative of the services being provided within the context of the interventions. The provision of outpatient treatment services, transportation and breakfast were highly appreciated by community members, both affected and non-affected alike. The following representative narratives attest to that.

*...for me the problem is that one cannot be admitted at the Obom clinic where we can go every morning and evening to attend to the patient and return to work on the farm. ...as soon as you go there, they will send you to Amasaman, which is very far away from here...very big town where you know nobody. ...once the child is on admission, you would have to remain with him as long as he stays at the hospital...your farm will be destroyed by rodents and weeds before you return. ...it is difficult to leave everything to go and stay at the hospital* (a mother of a patient, IDI at baseline).

*...sometimes you would want to go to the clinic but besides the money for transportation, you also find it difficult to leave other children at home because you are not sure that you will go on admission or you will be allowed to comeback. ...you have to go to the farm to bring home food for the family as foodstuff like cassava is better harvested on daily basis to avoid spoilage... but since the introduction of the free breakfast and transportation, it has*

*become easier for us to attend clinic as we do not have to worry about breakfast or transportation cost. ...one is able to go to farm or school after clinic attendance and this is good* (a mother of a patient, IDI at evaluation).

*...everybody is happy with how you are treating the BU patients now in our community. ...now, I do not have to go with my son to the clinic, all I have to do is make sure that he bathed and dressed for school....as he will be taken by the car free of charge and will be given food at the clinic..... taken to school on his way home... I can then take care of his father and siblings as well as go to the farm to work...* (mother of child with BU, IDI at evaluation).

BU victims, especially, children were stigmatized both at school and in the community and this was not only making them hide the infection but also drop out of school just to avoid being teased. However, with the community case searching and referral to the clinic, most of them were successfully treated and therefore could go to school without being stigmatized. The long hospital admission and the long times spent at hospital were also by themselves encouraging school dropout among the affected children. The interventions, especially transportation and feeding allowed children to receive treatment early at the clinic and return to school on a daily basis. The following narratives explained the situation at baseline and evaluation:

*...if you have this wound at school, people will laugh at you...you will not feel like going to school. When I first saw my wound (BU), I did not want anybody to know about it... not even my parents until it became very big and painful... I was afraid that my friends {would tease} me and that would make me stop going to school* (boy with BU, IDI at baseline).

*I am very happy to come to the clinic because I like the food that is given to us, especially the tea, which I don't normally drink at home... I sit in a car everyday and I like it very much...now when I go to school, I tell my friends about what I eat and how a car brought me to school... I also show them my wound and we are all happy that it was healing...now they no longer laugh at me and I am happy...* ( girl with BU, IDI at evaluation).

*...as you can see, at this place, we bring our foodstuffs home on daily basis, so if you miss going to the farm one day, it affects how much food you have at home... Most of our husbands work in the sand pit and are therefore paid on daily basis.... So it is difficult to leave other children who are healthy*

at home to starve… when you take one to the hospital only to be admitted and you cannot come home to take care of the rest including your husband (mother of an infected boy, IDI at baseline).

My child has been having this problem over three years ago… We did not go to the clinic because we were afraid that when we go, he will be hospitalized. …the current arrangement is good for us… I work in the sand pit…my wife works on the farm…it was difficult taking the child to the clinic but now the driver picks him every day to and from the hospital free of charge….who will not like this…? (father of boy with BU, IDI at evaluation).

I had this wound for some time now……I tried all forms of local herbs… sometimes it will look dry as if it was healing but it will not. I wanted to go to the clinic…the wound has become very big…getting vehicle to travel to the hospital was difficult. …I cannot walk on this leg to the hospital. Our roads are bad and no vehicle comes here, especially during the rainy season, even if a car managed to come, we cannot afford to go on daily basis …they charge so much…(affected young man, IDI at baseline).

…I think the best thing that has happened to us in this community is the provision of transportation to take BU patients to the clinic and back… we shall remain grateful and hope that you will continue to help us…to be free from this bad disease…so that our younger children will not suffer from it…I like the motorbike because it can go to every hamlet... (opinion leader, IDI at evaluation).

Our study focused on how to facilitate early case detection, diagnosis and treatment to reduce BU-related morbidity and disability. The social science literature on BU has tended to focus on perceptions and attitudes of local people to the infection, especially the clinical presentations, and the economic burden of disease to patients and their families.[6-8,10,12,13] Most studies that focus on finding cases were concerned only with referring them to the hospital where there was not enough space to accommodate all the cases referred, no accommodation for caretakers and very little consideration of the social effect of hospital admission on the affected families.[14] In the current study however, BU cases were treated on outpatient basis with no hospital admission. The provision of daily breakfast and transportation to the patients motivated them, especially children, not only to attend but endure taking injections daily for 56 continuous days. The provision of breakfast and transportation also afforded school children the opportunity to return to school on time and therefore reduced the motivation to stay away from school and consequently dropping out of school altogether.

Community case detection is not new in BU control in Ghana.[9] However, what makes this innovation unique is the outpatient treatment. The study attempted to address the five dimensions of access to health care,[17] by making sure that BU treatment services were available by training care providers on BU management including sample taking; and making basic supplies available to the health centre to ensure that they do not run out. Accessibility of the service was ensured through the provision of services at locations acceptable to patients, facilitated by free transport to carry patients to and from the clinic. Affordability was addressed by completely removing most of the indirect cost associated with treatment, as the cost of medication is covered by the state. Adequacy was addressed by making sure that services provided met the needs and expectations of patients by training and motivating providers to relate well to patients.

The number of cases referred by community-based volunteers increased significantly during the implementation of the intervention. This is attributable to the incentive schemes put in place to reward hardworking volunteers. The provision of bicycles for easy movement within the community did not lead to an increase in the number of cases referred in the first six month of implementation. However, when a token reward was introduced for hardworking individuals there was a significant increase in the number referred. This is an indication that we need to always find innovative ways to make volunteers feel rewarded for their services, even when we emphasize the voluntary nature of whatever they do. Especially when there are many persons involved, the hardworking ones should be recognized and appreciated as a way of encouraging them. Although, traditional healers did not contribute much in terms of the number of cases referred by them, we need to appreciate the symbolic meaning of them agreeing to collaborate with the health system to refer cases to the clinic as encouraging news that could be built upon in the future.

The interventions implemented in this study could not have been made without cost implications but this should not be exaggerated. In the long run, it may be cheaper to implement these activities to diagnose and treat patients early as outpatients than to receive them late into the health system where they will have to be managed with surgery and require long-term hospitalisation in most cases. Affected persons (i.e. patients and their family caretakers) complained of long hospital stay as one of the reasons why they do not usually attend hospital because of the social costs (leaving other family members behind, leaving farm work behind, which usually led to the destruction of farms in their absence, etc.) that came with hospital admissions. BU affects mostly the poorest of the poor and this should be enough motivation for implementing interventions to reduce the disease burden on this vulnerable population. However, there is a need for a cost-benefit analysis of the interventions implemented in this study for a better appreciation of what it will take to scale up the intervention.

## Conclusion

It was clear from the study that providing breakfast and free transport to patients contributed significantly to the near elimination of treatment default and dropout among patients. Thus, with a little more investment in early case detection, diagnosis and treatment, coupled with free transportation and breakfast for patients, most BU cases could be treated effectively with the available antibiotics to avoid and / or reduce disabilities due to the disease. It is therefore worth the investment to support the poorest of the poor in remote villages to access health care to avoid disability due to BU and also keep children in school when receiving effective treatment for Buruli ulcer.

## Acknowledgements

Our thanks go to the Ga South Municipal health administration, especially the staff of Obom health centre for fruitful collaboration. We thank the chiefs and people of the study communities for their support. We thank the volunteers, traditional healers and former patients for implementing the interventions. Thanks go to the respondents for agreeing to participate in the study without which there would be no study. Mr. Isaac Lamptey and Mr. Seth Baffoe deserve special mention for leading the outreach activities. Financial support was provided by the Optimus Foundation, UBS through the Stop Buruli Consortium, Switzerland.

# References

1. Van der Werf, T. S., Stienstra, Y., Johnson, R.C. *et al.* (2005) *Mycobacterium ulcerans disease. Bull.* WHO 83: 785–791.
2. World Health Organization (2008) Buruli ulcer: progress report, 2004-2008. *Wkly Epidemiol Rec* 83: 145–154.
3. Johnson, P. D., Stinear, T., Small, P. L., Pluschke, G., Merritt, R.W., Portaels, F., Huygen, K., Hayman, J. A., and Asiedu, K. (2005) Buruli ulcer (M. ulcerans infection): new insights, new hope for disease control. *PLoS. Med.* 2: e108.
4. Sizaire V, Nackers F, Comte E, Portaels F. (2006) *Mycobacterium ulcerans* infection: control, diagnosis, and treatment. *The Lancet Infectious Diseases* 6: 288–296. doi: 10.1016/S1473-3099(06) 70464-9.
5. Amofa, G., Bonsu, F., Tetteh, C., Okrah, J., Asamoah, K., Asiedu, K. and Addy, J. (2002). Buruli ulcer in Ghana: Results of a national case search. *Emerging Infectious Diseases*, 8: 167-170
6. Adamba, C. and Owusu, A. Y. (2011). Burden of Buruli Ulcer: How affected households in a Ghanaian district cope. *African Study Monographs,* 32: 1-23.
7. Peeters Grietens, K., Um Boock, A., Peeters, H., Hausmann-Muela, S., Toomer, E. *et al.* (2008) "It Is Me Who Endures but My Family That Suffers": Social Isolation as a Consequence of the Household Cost Burden of Buruli Ulcer Free of Charge Hospital Treatment. *PLoS Negl Trop Dis* 2: e321.doi: 10.1371/ journal.pntd.0000321.
8. Renzaho Andre, M. N., Woods Paul, V., Ackumey, Mercy M., Harvey Simon, K. and Kotin Jacob. (2007) Community-based study on knowledge, attitude and practice on the mode of transmission, prevention and treatment of the Buruli ulcer in Ga West District, Ghana. *Trop Med and Int Health:* 12, 445–458.
9. Debacker, M., Aguiar, J., Steunou, C., Zinsou, C., Meyers, W.M, et al. (2004) Mycobacterium ulcerans disease: role of age and gender

in incidence and morbidity. *Trop Med Int Health* 9: 1297–1304. doi:10.1111/j.1365- 3156.2004.01339.x.

10. Aujoulat, I., Johnson, C., Zinsou, C., Gue´de´non, A. and Portaels F. (2003) Psychosocial aspects of health seeking behaviours of patients with Buruli ulcer in southern Benin. *Tropical Medicine and International Health:* 8, 750–759

11. Stienstra, Y., van der Graaf, W. T., Asamoa, K. and van der Werf, T.S. (2002) Beliefs and attitudes toward Buruli ulcer in Ghana. *Am J Trop Med Hyg* 67:207–213.

12. Bigelow, J., Welling ,R., Sinnott, R. and Evenson, R. (2002) Attitudes toward clinical and traditional treatment for Buruli ulcer in the Ga district, Ghana. *Annals Af Med* 1, 99-111.

13. Asiedu, K. and Etuaful, S .(1998) Socioeconomic implications of Buruli ulcer in Ghana: a three-year review. *Am J Trop Med Hyg* 59: 1015-1022

14. Ackumey, M. M., Kwakye-Maclean, C., Ampadu, E. O., de Savigny, D., Weiss, M. G. (2011) Health services for Buruli ulcer control: Lessons from a field study in Ghana. *PLoS Negl Trop Dis* 5(6): e1187. doi:10.1371/journal.pntd.0001187.

15. Farmer, P. (1999) Infections and Inequalities: The Modern Plagues. Berkeley: University of California Press.

16. Etuaful, S., Carbonnelle, B., Grosset, J., Lucas, S., Horsfield, C., et al. Efficacy of the combination rifampin-streptomycin in preventing growth of Mycobacterium ulcerans in early lesions of Buruli ulcer in humans (2005). *Antimicrob Agents Chemother* 49: 3182–3186.

17. Obrist, B., Iteba, N., Lengeler, C., Makemba, A., Mshana, C., et al. (2007) Access to health care in contexts of livelihood insecurity: A framework for analysis and action. *PLoS Med* 4(10): e308. doi:10.1371/journal.pmed.0040308.

# Chapter 14
## Poly-parasitism of *Plasmodium Falciparum* and Helminths Among School Children in Three Peri-urban Communities in Ghana

*Irene Ayi, Ato Kwamena Tetteh, Joseph Otchere, Langbong Bimi, Daniel Adjei Boakye*

## Introduction

*Plasmodium falciparum* is known to occur in association with intestinal helminths (*Ascaris lumbricoides*, *Trichuris trichiura* and hookworms), which infect more than a third of Africans.[1] The schistosomes, *Schistosoma haematobium* and *S. mansoni*, are also endemic throughout Africa and associate with *P. falciparum*, but generally have a much more focal distribution than intestinal helminth species.[2] Co-infections of helminths have been extensively documented, and occur as a result of similar life cycle and modes of infection as well as suitable environmental factors and human practices which support the survival of these parasites. Interactions between *P. falciparum* and different helminths are not well understood. Preliminary analyses elsewhere suggest that as many as one quarter of African school children may be coincidentally at risk of *P. falciparum* and hookworm co-infections.[3] Poly-parasitism involving these two parasites is particularly common, although the public health significance of poly-parasitic infection remains unclear. The pathology due to co-infection of *Plasmodium* species and helminths is significant, due to blood and nutrient loss, resulting in anaemia, which impact negatively on growth and cognitive development of school-aged children.

According to studies conducted in malaria-endemic populations in Africa, helminth infections have been reported to increase susceptibility to clinical malaria,[4,5] reduce the risk[6] or make no difference.[7] Studies in Thailand also suggest that helminth infections might increase the risk of non-severe malaria, but reduce the risk of cerebral malaria.[8,9] The ability of worms to shift the immune response toward $Th_2$ cytokines is well established.[10] The $Th_2$ cytokine milieu induced by helminth infection is thought to drive the antibody response of malaria co-infected individuals towards the production of non-cytophilic subclasses ($IgG_2$, $IgG_4$, and IgM), whereas protection against malaria is associated with the presence of the $IgG_1$ and $IgG_3$ cytophilic subclasses.[11,12] The cytokine milieu could also favour either pro- or anti-inflammatory reactions during malaria infection.[13] Information on associations and mechanisms linked to co-infection of *P. falciparum* and helminths in Ghana is limited, although the public health implication is high. The purpose of this study was to investigate the existence of multi-infection with *Plasmodium sp., Schistosoma sp.* and intestinal helminths in at risk Ghanaian children.

# Approach

## Study area

The study was conducted in Kasseh, Ghana, a peri-urban area 100 km east of Accra. This area is typically coastal savanna, characterized by dry climatic conditions with the smallest amount of rainfall in Ghana. Two annual rainfall peaks (April to June and September to October) for the area range between 740-900 mm of rain. The highest mean monthly temperature is 30°C (March-April), and the lowest 26°C (August). Relative humidity is high throughout the year, and it ranges between 65-80%. Crop farming in the area is mainly for cash and subsistence, especially, the growing of fruits such as mangoes and watermelons and vegetables, including tomatoes and pepper. There are also piggeries and cattle ranches.

## Study population

The study population consisted of children from three primary schools living in three villages (Afiadenyigba, Dorgobom and Tojeh) in the Dangme East District. Although the assumed age range of pupils in primary schools in Ghana is 6 to 12 years, the situation is different in rural areas, including our study population.

## Sample size

Assuming a 95% confidence interval and average parasitic diseases prevalence of 60%, a minimum sample size of 369 pupils was needed. A total of 381 pupils aged 3 to 26 years (which includes the age group at risk), were sampled on voluntary basis after informed consent.

## Study design

The study was cross-sectional and was conducted from July to October 2007. Personal data were recorded for all participants. In addition, questionnaire interviews about their knowledge of transmission of malaria and helminthiasis was administered. Investigations for malaria status of participants included examination and interview for uncomplicated signs and symptoms, as well as microscopic examination of capillary blood smears for malaria parasites. Stool and urine samples were also obtained for microscopic detection of parasites' ova.

Approval and ethical clearance was obtained from the STC and IRB of the NMIMR (CPN 038/06-07) after which informed consent was sought from the school and health authorities, parents and guardians with the children assenting.

## Questionnaire survey and data collection

Questionnaires on personal information were self-administered by the upper primary pupils after explanation in a local language by the teachers and local field workers, whilst lower primary children were interviewed. The questions included age, sex and other relevant information on their knowledge of exposure to infection risk factors and treatment history for malaria, schistosomiasis and intestinal helminthiasis. Explanations were made in a manner that enabled pupils to provide appropriate answers without influencing their choices. Pupils were questioned and examined for the presence of shivers, chills, headaches and fever by taking axillary temperature using a digital thermometer and recorded for three consecutive days before finger-prick blood collection. The definition for uncomplicated malaria in this study was based on the criteria as defined by the Ghana Malaria Policy Document.[14] The three main symptoms; fever, chills, and shivering and/or headache were observed over a three-day period, with fever defined as an axillary temperature of ≥37.5°C

## Collection and analysis of biological samples

Thick and thin blood films were prepared from finger-prick blood on appropriately labelled glass microscope slides (25 x 75 mm). Giemsa staining was done following fixing of the thin blood films in methanol. Stained blood films were examined under 100 magnification with oil immersion. *Plasmodium* species identification was based on the morphology of the various life stages. Malaria parasites identified were counted per 200 leucocytes and converted to the number of parasites per µL of blood, assuming a leucocyte count of 8000/µL of blood as a standard, to estimate the intensity of infection. Appropriately labelled screw cap containers were given to pupils to produce urine for collection between the hours of 10:00 and 15:00, when egg excretion is known to be highest.[15] The samples were transported in a cool box to the laboratory for processing and examination within six hours of collection. A graduated syringe was used to draw 10 ml out of each total urine specimen after thorough mixing. The urine was then filtered through the polycarbon membrane (diameter 25 mm; pore size 12.0 µm; Nucleopore, Track-Etch) fitted in the assembled filtration apparatus. Air was pushed through the apparatus with the aid of the syringe to remove excess urine. The nucleopore filter membranes were removed and placed face down on appropriately labelled glass microscope slides which were examined under the microscope with low magnification. Air-dried membranes on slides were packed into slide boxes and examined later. To improve the refractive index for dried membranes during examination, a drop of normal saline was placed at the edge of the membrane at one side and allowed to wet the surface.[15] Schistosome eggs were identified and counted. Intensity of infection was recorded as eggs per 10 ml of urine.[16]

Stool samples from the pupils were collected in well labelled sterile specimen containers with screw lids provided them prior to the day of collection with clear instructions. Each pupil provided about 3 to 5g of their early morning stool which were transported in a cool box to the laboratory, stored at 4°C, processed and examined within 2 weeks using the Kato-Katz method.[17] Briefly, a portion of stool sample was sieved through a nylon mesh with pore size of 105 μm. Part of the sieved specimen was taken to fill a hole (diameter: 7 mm) in the card template set on a glass microscope slide. The intact plug of stool on the slide (0.027g) was covered with a cellophane cover slip (29 x 35 mm treated with 50% (v/v) glycerol in water containing 3% malachite green) after removal of the template. The slide was turned upside down on the flat working surface and pressed to spread the stool evenly under the cover slip, left in a dust-free area for up to 30 min at room temperature and examined microscopically to detect intestinal parasites' eggs. Parasites eggs detected were identified morphologically, counted and the number of eggs counted in each stool sample was multiplied by a factor of 37 (i.e. 1/0.027g) to estimate the eggs per gram (epg) of faeces. This was used to classify *S. mansoni* and soil-transmitted helminth infections based on the WHO criteria (2002)[16] as light, moderate or high intensity.

## Data Analysis

Data were entered by two independent data entry clerks, cleaned in Microsoft Excel,™ and exported to SPSS 12.0 for descriptive statistical analyses, including the estimation of the prevalence and intensity of parasite infections. Prevalence of *P. falciparum* and helminth co-infection among age groups was also determined. Differences between categorical variables were tested by the chi squad test.

## Results

A total of 381 pupils aged 3 to 26 years (sd+ = 3.4) from three primary schools participated in the study. They comprised of 199 (52.2%) males and 182 (47.8%) females. The age group generally considered to be at high risk of parasitic infections, especially worms (8-12 year olds), constituted 195/381 (51.2%). They comprised of 26 (6.8%) of ≤ 6 years, 95 (24.9%) 7-9 years, 127 (33.3%) 10-12 years, 90 (23.6%) 13-15 years, 35 (9.2%) 16-18 years and 8 (2.1%) ≥ 19 years age groups. Ninety-eight percent (374/381) of the pupils were between the ages of 7 and 18, while those with extreme ages outside this age group constituted 7/381 (1.8%). There was no significant difference between the prevalence among males and females ($\chi^2$ = 2.037, p = 0.096) and among the age groups as well ($\chi^2$ = 4.806, p = 0.440).

Six parasites were detected among the pupils as follows: *P. falciparum* (*Pf*) 81/381, *S. haematobium* (*Sh*) 76/381, hookworms (*Hw*) 53/381, *T. trichiura* (*Tt*) 12/381, *S. mansoni* (*Sm*) 4/381 and *Hymenelopis nana* (*Hn*) 1/381 (Table 14.1). Overall, 176/381 (46.2%) of the pupils were found to be infected with at least one parasite. Single parasite infection was found among 129/381 (33.9%) of the pupils and included *P. falciparum* (12.9%), *S. haematobium* (11.5%), hookworms (7.1%), *T. trichiura* (1.8%) and *S. mansoni* (0.5%).

Table14. 1:   Prevalence of parasitic infections among schools

| Commu-nity school | Parasites detected n (%) | | | | | |
|---|---|---|---|---|---|---|
| | *P. falci-parum* | *S. haema-tobium* | Hook-worm | *T. trichiura* | *S. mansoni* | *H. nana* |
| Afiade-nyigba (AF) | 67 (17.6) | 29 (7.6) | 37 (9.7) | 4 (1.0) | 2 (0.5) | 1 (0.3) |
| Dorgobom (DB) | 13 (3.4) | 14 (3.7) | 1 (0.3) | 3 (0.8) | 1 (0.3) | - |
| Tojer (TJ) | 1 (0.3) | 33 (8.7) | 15 (3.9) | 5 (1.3) | 1 (0.3) | - |
| Total prevalence (%) | 81 (21.3) | 76 (19.9) | 53 (13.9) | 12 (3.1) | 4 (1.0) | 1 (0.3) |

The, prevalence of *P. falciparum* was significantly higher among the high risk group (8-12) compared to $\leq$ 7 years age group (p<0.05) but insignificant compared with the $\geq$ 13 years age group (p>0.05) [Figure14.1]. There was also no significant difference in *S. haematobium* and hookworm infections among the age groups considered (Figure14.1).

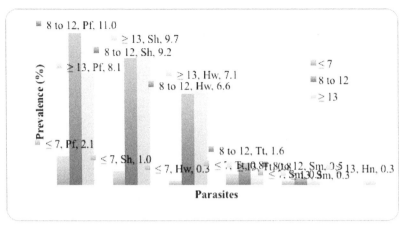

*Figure 14.1: Prevalence of parasitic infections among age groups*

*Pf* = *Plasmodium falciparum*; *Sh* = *Schistosoma haematobium*;
*Hw* = *Hookworms*; *Tt* = *Trichuris trichiura*; *Sm* = *S. mansoni*; *Hn* = *Hymenolepis nana*

## *P. falciparum* and helminth co-infection

Ten multiple infection combinations (*Pf/Hw, Pf/Sh, Pf/Tt, Pf/Sh/Hn, Pf/Sh/Hw, Pf/Sh/Tt, Sh/Hw, Sh/Sm, Sh/Tt, Hw/Tt*), were found among 47/381 (12.3%) of the pupils. Forty-three of these (91.5%) were infected with two different parasites each, while the remaining 4 were infected with three. Thirty-three of the 47 (70.2%) involved *P. falciparum*, which is 6 out of the 10 multiple infection combinations, as follows *Pf/Hw, Pf/Sh, Pf/Tt, Pf/Sh/Hn, Pf/Sh/Hw, Pf/Sh/Tt*. [Figure 14.2].

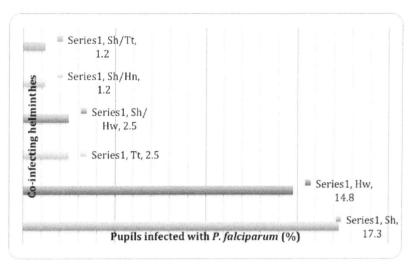

Figure 14.2: Prevalence of *P. falciparum* and co-infecting helminths

*Sh = Schistosoma haematobium; Hw = Hookworms; Tt = Trichuris trichiura;*
*Sm = S. mansoni; Hn = Hymenolepis nana*

Plasmodium falciparum was detected in 81 pupils and there was no difference in parasite density among the age groups. Out of these, 33 (40.7%) were additionally infected with helminths (Table14.2). Thirty-one of these were of low intensity and in combination with low-intensity helminth infections as well. Moderate intensity of *P. falciparum* infection was detected among two pupils in the 10-12 years age group who were also infected with *S. haematobium* and hookworms in low intensities. There was no significant difference in *P. falciparum* infection intensity among males and females p = 0.336) or among age groups p = 0.633)

Table 14.2: Prevalence and distribution of *P. falciparum* with single and multi-helminth infection intensities among age groups

| Intensity of *P. falciparum* | Age group (yrs) | Single helminthes %(n) | | | | Multi-helminthes %(n) | | | Total |
|---|---|---|---|---|---|---|---|---|---|
| | | | S. haematobium | Hookworms | T. trichiura | Sh/Hw | Sh/Tt | Sh/Hn | |
| | | (1-9)*[b] | (10-49)[g][b] | (1-1999)*[c] | (1-999)*[c] | | | | |
| Low (40-4999)[a] | 7-9 | 6.1 (2) | - | 15.2(5) | 3.0 (1) | - | - | - | 24.2(8) |
| | 10-12 | - | 3.0(1) | 3.0(1) | - | - | 3.0 (1) | - | 9.1(3) |
| | 13-15 | 12.1 (4) | 6.1 (2) | 9.1 (3) | - | 3.0 (1) | - | 3.0(1) | 33.3 (11) |
| | 16-18 | 9.1(3) | 3.0 (1) | 6.1(2) | 3.0 (1) | - | - | - | 21.2 (7) |
| | ≥19 | 3.0 (1) | - | - | - | 3.0 (1 | - | - | 6.1(2) |
| Moderate (5000-99999)[a] | 10-12 | - | 3.0 (1 | 3.0 (1) | - | - | - | - | 6.1(2) |
| Total | | 30.3 (10) | 15.2 (5) | 36.4 (12) | 6.1 (2) | 6.1 (2) | 3.0 (1) | 3.0 (1) | (33) |

The intensity of *P. falciparum* infections ranged from light to moderate, with counts between 40 and 23,360 parasites /µL of blood. Infection intensity of all other parasites detected were light. Number of pupils infected with *P. falciparum* decreased with increasing number of co-infecting helminth species (Table 14.2). Mean axillary temperatures over three days for pupils with *P. falciparum*-helminth co-infections ranged between 35.8 and 37.0°C. Of the 81, 27 (33.3%) had chills/rigors or headache for two to three consecutive days.

## KAP

In all, 373 (97.9%) pupils responded to a questionnaire on their practices and general information about some common parasitic diseases (malaria, schistosomiasis and soil-transmitted helminthiasis). Out of this number, 288 (77.2%) responded as having been previously infected with intestinal helminthes, *Schistosoma haematobium,* 159 (42.6%) with *S. mansoni* and 251 (67.3%) with *Plasmodium* sp. In all, 103 (27.6%) pupils lived in houses close to potential breeding/hiding grounds of mosquitoes. Most of the respondents mentioned the following control measures; weeding, 310 (83.1%), burning/burying of refuse, 287 (76.9%) and cleaning choked gutters, (218) 58.4%. Of the 373, 48.5% experienced mosquito bites. Many pupils, 245 (66.2%), indicated that they slept under bednets to avoid mosquito bites, 158 (42.3%) and 1 (0.3%), used untreated bednets. Fewer pupils used insect repellents/insecticides, trap doors and windows, or burned particular weeds as mosquito repellents.

Respondents 274 (73.5%) indicated that they had experienced various signs/symptoms of uncomplicated malaria (i.e. chills/rigors/fever/headache) while 60 (16.1%) had none in the six months before the survey. Less than 40% of pupils (145) indicated contact with freshwater bodies within their communities. Also 275 (73.7%) had come into contact with a fresh water body outside their communities, to fetch water, bathe and/or play games and catch fish. Overall, 336 (90.1%) pupils accompanied their parents to farm/garden, while 157 (42.1%) accompanied parents to fish in a water body. One hundred and forty four 144 (59.8%) pupils had experienced bloody urine and painful micturition. Similarly, 84 (22.5%) indicated having ever experienced swollen stomach and bloody stool. Responses related to soil-transmitted helminthiasis (STH) infection. Approximately, 80% of pupils put on footwere at home and at school; but most of them (58.7%)removed them while at play. The majority of pupils used KVIP at home (69.2%) and at school (82.3) as a place of convenience. Almost a quarter of the pupils (25.7%) indicated using open spaces.

## Discussion

Poly-parasitism in humans is of particular public health concern due to their potential of causing diverse debilitating disease pathologies, especially in children of school-going age. Many studies have reported the susceptibility of malaria-infected individuals to helminths infection in most developing countries[4,5,6,7] but published data on the issue in Ghana is limited. Therefore, this study was conducted to assess the situation in school-age children in a peri-urban area in Ghana. *Plasmodium falciparum, S. haematobium* and hookworm infections were the most prevalent in the study participants. Parasites detected did not include *A. lumbricoides*, which triggers immunologic responses that, according to Murrey *et al.*,[18] were known to down-regulate the growth and multiplication of *Plasmodium* sp. In another study they observed the relative absence of malaria in children with heavy *A. lumbricoides* infection, and a remarkable recrudescence of malaria following treatment of these children,[19] leading to the postulation that nutritional consequences of severe ascariasis led to malaria suppression in order to maintain host survival. However, a later study found a positive correlation between helminths and *Plasmodium sp* co-infection.[20] The high prevalence of *P. falciparum* found in this study could be attributed to the absence of *A. lumbricoides*. Non-detection of *A. lumbricoides*, however, does not rule out the possibility of it being present in the communities. The remaining parasites infecting the pupils together with *P. falciparum* were found in too few of the pupils to make any meaningful statistical analysis. However, they are of as much public health importance as the more prevalent parasites.

Particular note was taken of *S. haematobium* infection among age groups and sex since differences have been reported. Effects of age and sex on infection with schistosomiasis are well known and are associated with the type and number of water contacts. Results in this study diverge from earlier reports that boys are much more infected with *S. haematobium* as they take more baths.[21,22,23] This study found no significant difference (p > 0.05) among age groups and sexes for both *S. haematobium* and other parasites detected.

The risk of exposure to infection with *P. falciparum, S. haematobium* and hookworm was high. Although we did not ascertain the use of night soil in either commercial or subsistence farming in communities, pupils responded to using open spaces as places of convenience. It is typical that these children only put on footwear when going to school, and even remove them when playing outdoors. About 60% of pupils removed their footwear during play at school and at home, usually for comfort or to avoid the risk of early wear and tear. It was common to find both children and adults in the communities going barefooted. With the presence of these risks of exposure to parasitic infections, children are likely to be infected with more than one of the three main parasites detected. Water contact was confirmed by responses to the questionnaire, with 73.7% of pupils affirming having freshwater contact within or outside their communities. Majority of these children indicated being involved in water contact activities such as bathing and playing in freshwater bodies. Even though 66.2% of the children indicated using mosquito nets, they also admitted playing at night before going to sleep under their nets. The risk was high as more than 80% of them indicated being bitten by mosquitoes at evening/dusk and night. It was observed that the household compounds in the study villages had bushy backyards and used uncovered water pots containing water that was fetched from nearby ponds and streams. The exposure to infection risk factors, however, did not culminate in infection with the associated parasites.

Children aged 8 to 12 years are involved in the collection of biological data for prevalence/incidence estimation of helminthiasis for the planning of disease control programmes in schools and communities. This age group formed the highest proportion, 195/381 (51.2%), of participants in this study. The inclusion of so-called 'outliers' (aged < 8 and > 12 years) in this study could be of signifi-cance in the planning and implementation of school-based disease control programmes in rural and peri-urban settings, especially in Africa. Individuals in the same class though of different ages could be involved in similar activities which may result in similar infection patterns. Such activities may involve playing in school and/or home as well as visiting potentially contaminated sites such as water bodies, refuse dumps and farms where human and animal excreta is used as manure. Findings made in this study bring to the fore, the importance of screening all pupils, regardless of age, in rural and peri-urban areas in Ghana.

Individuals with multiple parasite infections were all in the light intensity range with the respective parasites. Similar studies in Senegal[23] showed that children lightly infected with *S. haematobium* had lower *P. falciparum* densities than the uninfected, suggesting a negative interaction between both parasites. Furthermore, studies in Mali[6] showed no association between *P. falciparum* and *S. haematobium*. These are contrary to recent studies[2] which revealed an association between the two parasites.

Most pupils were infected with *P. falciparum, S. haematobium* and hookworm. All these three parasites cause anaemia and growth retardation through the loss of blood and nutrients.[17] *Plasmodium falciparum* especially contributes to reducing haemoglobin concentration through a number of mechanisms. Principal amongst them is the destruction and removal of parasitized erythrocytes, shortening of the life span of non-parasitized erythrocytes and decreasing the rate of erythrocyte production in the bone marrow. Infection with hookworm results in iron deficiency anaemia through intestinal blood loss. Schistosomes also contribute to anaemia by chronic blood loss as eggs penetrate the wall of the bowels and urinary bladder. Infection with helminths in general could result in under-nutrition with or without anaemia. Both conditions are commonly reported in *T. trichiura* infections,[24] which results in rectal prolapse with high intensities.

The primary setback of co-infections studies is whether observations made mainly in animal models under controlled conditions are applicable in human populations. This is especially important to establish since infected individuals presented virtually no symptoms. Further detailed studies will be significant for understanding of the immunological mechanisms and public health implications of co-infections in Ghana. Nationwide mass drug administration in Ghana have so far concentrated on neglected tropical diseases, notably, schistosomiasis, lymphatic filariasis and intestinal helminths using appropriate broad-spectrum anthelmintics, either alone or in combination. Such integrated control programmes target several parasitic worm infections simultaneously except for malaria. In *P. falciparum*-helminth-infected individuals, these programmes could only avert both immediate and long-term morbidities due to multi-parasitic worm infections in individuals, especially among children of school-going age. School-age children with *Plasmodium* sp. parasitaemia tend to serve as reservoir for malaria transmission but malaria control interventions focus on infants less than 5 years old and pregnant women. Intensive malaria-related activities in schools[25] and integration of educative information on malaria in textbooks will go a long way towards effective school-based malaria control.[26]

## Conclusion

This study provides evidence of poly-parasitism in school-age children. Integrated worm control programmes targeting multiple parasitic worm infestations in school-age children could include malaria control to avert deleterious consequences due to parasite co-infections.

## References

1.  Brooker, S., Clements, A., C. A., Bundy, D. A. P. Global epidemiology, ecology and control of soil-transmitted helminth infections. *Adv Parasitol* (2006a) 62: 221–261.
2.  Brooker, S. Spatial epidemiology of human schistosomiasis in Africa: risk models, transmission dynamics and control. *Trans R Soc Trop Med Hyg* (2007)101: 1–8.
3.  Brooker, S., Clements, A. C., Hotez, P. J., Hay, S. I., Tatem, A. J., Bundy, D. A., Snow R. W. The co-distribution of *Plasmodium falciparum* and hookworms among African schoolchildren. *Malaria J* (2006 b) 5: 99.

4.  Spiegel, A., Tall. A., Raphenon, G., Trape, J. F., Druilhe, P. Increased frequency of malaria attacks in subjects co-infected by intestinal worms and *Plasmodium falciparum* malaria. *Trans R Soc Trop Med Hyg* (2003) 97: 198–199.

5.  Sokhna, C., Le Hesran, J. Y., Mbaye, P. A., Akiana, J., Camara, P. Increase of malaria attacks among children presenting concomitant infection by *Schistosoma mansoni* in Senegal. *Malaria J* (2004) 3: 43.

6.  Lyke, K. E., Dicko, A., Dabo, A., Sangare, L., Kone, A. Association of *Schistosoma haematobium* infection with protection against acute *Plasmodium falciparum* malaria in Malian children. *Am J Trop Med Hyg* (2005) 73: 1124–1130.

7.  Shapiro, A. E., Tukahebwa, E. M., Kasten, J., Clarke, S. E., Magnussen, P. Epidemiology of helminth infections and their relationship to clinical malaria in southwest Uganda. *Trans R Soc Trop Med Hyg* (2005) 99: 18–24.

8.  Nacher, M., Gay, F., Singhasivanon, P., Krudsood, S., Treeprasertsuk, S. *Ascaris lumbricoides* infection is associated with protection from cerebral malaria. *Parasite Immunol* (2000) 22: 107–113.

9.  Nacher, M. Malaria vaccine trials in a wormy world. *Trends Parasitol* (2001) 17: 563–565.

10. Bentwich, Z., Weisman, Z., Moroz, C., Bar-Yehuda, S., Kalinkovich, A. Immune disregulation in Ethiopian immigrants in Israel: relevance to helminth infections? *Clin Exp Immunol* (1996) 103: 239-243.

11. Druilhe, P., Tall, A. Worms can worsen malaria: towards a new means to roll back malaria? *Trends Parasitol* (2005) 21: 359–362.

12. Sridhar, V., Basavaraju, M. D., Peter Schantz, V. M. D. Soil-Transmitted helminths and *Plasmodium falciparum* malaria: Epidemiology, Clinical Manifestations, and the Role of Nitric Oxide in Malaria and Geohelminth Co-infection. Do Worms Have a Protective Role in *P. falciparum* Infection? *The Mount Sinai J Med* (2006). 73: 8.

13. Diallo, T. O., Remoue, F., Schacht, A. M., Charrier, N., Dompnier, J. P. Schistosomiasis co-infection in humans influences inflammatory markers in uncomplicated *Plasmodium falciparum* malaria. *Parasite Immunol* (2004) 26: 365–369.

14. Ghana Health Service (2004) Guidelines for Case Management of Malaria in Ghana.

15. Peters, P. A. Rapid accurate quantification of schistosome eggs via nucleopore filters. *J Parasitol* (1976) 62: 154-155.

16. WHO (World Health Organization). *Prevention and Control of Schistosomiasis and Soil-Transmitted Helminthiasis.* Geneva: World Health Organization; 2002. *WHO Tech Ser Rep* (2002) 912 pp.
17. Mupfasoni, D., Karibushi, B., Koukounari, A., Ruberanziza, E., Kaberuka, T., Kramer, M. H., Mukabayire, O., Kabera, M., Nizeyimana, V., Deville, M., Ruxin, J., Joanne, P. Polyparasite helminth infections and their association to anaemia and undernutrition in Northern Rwanda. *J PLoS NTD* (2009) 3(9): e517. doi:10.1371/journal.pntd.0000517
18. Murray, M. J., Murray, A. B., Murray, M. B., Murray, C. J. Parotid enlargement, forehead oedema, and suppression of malaria as nutritional consequences of ascariasis. *Am J Clin Nutrit* (1977) 30 (12): 2117–2121.
19. Murray, M. J., Murray, A. B., Murray, M. B., Murray, C. J. The biological suppression of malaria: an ecological and nutritional interrelationship of a host and two parasites. *Am J Clin Nutrit* (1978) 31 (8): 1363–1366.
20. Tshikuka, J. G., Scott, M. E., Gray-Donald, K., Kalumba, O. N. Multiple infection with *Plasmodium* and helminths in communities of low and relatively high socio-economic status. *Ann Trop Med Parasitol* (1996) 90 (3): 277–293.
21. Woolhouse, M. E. J., Watts, C. H., Chandiwana, S. K. Heterogeneities in transmission rates and the epidemiology of schistosome infection. *Proc R Soc Lond B Biol Sci* (1991) 245:109–114.
22. Chandiwana, S. K. and Woolhouse, M. E. J. Heterogeneities in water contacts patterns and the epidemiology of *Schistosoma haematobium*. *Parasitology* (1991) 103: 363–370.
23. Briand, V. R., Watier, L., Le Hesran, J. Y., Garcia, A., Cot, M. Co-infection with *Plasmodium falciparum* and *Schistosoma haematobium*: Protective effect of schistosomiasis on malaria in Senegalese children? *Am J Trop Med Hyg* (2005) 72(6): 702–707.
24. Bundy, D. A. P. Cooper, E. S. *Trichuris* and trichuriasis in humans. *Adv Parasitol* (1989) 28: 107–173.
25. Ayi, I., Nonaka, D., Adjovu, J. K., Hanafusa, S., Jimba, M., Bosompem, K. M., Mizoue, T., Takeuchi, T., Boakye D. A., Kobayashi, J. School-based participatory health education for malaria control in Ghana: engaging children as health messengers. *Malaria J* (2010) 9: 98 http://www.malariajournal.com/content/9/1/98.
26. Nonaka, D., Jimba, M., Mizoue, T., Kobayashi, J., Yasuoka, J., Ayi, I., Silva, A. C., Shrestha, S., Kikuchi, K., Haque, S. E., Yi, S. Analysis of primary and secondary school textbooks regarding malaria control:

a multi-country study *PLoS ONE* (2011) 7(5): e36629. Doi:10.1371/ journal.pone.003662.

# Chapter 15
# Towards Unravelling the Complexities of Filarial Diseases Transmission and Research for Control in Ghana

*Dziedzom K. de Souza, Daniel A. Boakye and Michael D. Wilson*

## Introduction

Lymphatic filariasis (LF), commonly known as elephantiasis is a neglected tropical disease, prevalent in wide areas of the African continent. It is caused by infection with the filarial parasites *Wuchereria bancrofti*, *Brugiamalayi* and *Brugiatimori*.[1] It is transmitted through the bites of infective female mosquito vectors belonging to the genera *Anopheles*, *Culex*, *Mansonia* and *Aedes*, depending on the geographic region. In West Africa, *An. gambiae*sensu lato and *An. funestus* group are the most important vectors.

The disease is profoundly disfiguring, and is one of the leading causes of permanent disability in the world. The most common clinical manifestation of LF is the lymphoedema of the legs and genitalia.[1] The disease has been targeted for elimination by the Global Programme for Elimination of Lymphatic Filariasis (GPELF) by 2020.[2] The elimination strategy is mass drug administration (MDA), through a yearly combination treatment with albendazole (ALB) and diethyl-carbamazine (DEC), or albendazole and ivermectin – depending on the epidemiologic situation – to all at-risk populations in endemic areas. It is envisaged that such a strategy will control morbidity and eventually reduce microfilaraemia (mf) long enough for it to fall to levels at which transmission cannot be sustained. The early LF parasitological and epidemiological studies conducted in Ghana, especially in communities along the coastal areas[3,4,5] and in the northern sections of the country[6] involved scientists from the NMIMR. Dunyo and colleagues[3] showed that there was little or no LF in villages east of

Accra. However, high LF prevalence was observed in coastal villages west of Accra.

Entomology studies identified *An. gambiae* s.l. and *An. funestus-*group as the major vectors of the disease.[3,6] Dzodzomenyo and colleagues[5] showed that the abundance of these vectors and their relative importance vary considerably between the wet and the dry seasons. Recent studies revealed that *Culex* and *Aedes* were not vectors of LF in Ghana[7] but rather *Mansonia species* were very effective vectors.[8] Other studies focused on the vector-parasite interactions all aimed at understanding the transmission dynamics in different areas.[9,10,11,12]

In West Africa, it is believed that the *Anopheles* vectors exhibit "facilitation"– a process which describes situations in which the vectors are unable to transmit the disease at low microfilaraemia levels in human population. However, studies by Boakye *et al.*[9] Clement[10] and Amuzu *et al.*[11] showed that in some areas of Ghana the vectors exhibit "limitation"– where the vectors are efficient and are able to transmit at low microfilaraemia levels. Despite these various studies, an enigma that begs for an explanation is why LF endemicity is restricted to northern and southern Ghana, with the middle belt free of the disease,[13] whilst the known LF vectors are the same ones that transmit malaria which is endemic throughout the country. We therefore conducted a study to seek an explanation hypothesizing that environmental factors and genetic differences within and between both *An. gambiae s.s.* and *W. bancrofti* are responsible for the observed distribution pattern.

# Approach

Biting mosquitoes were collected off human bait at 14 sites in four ecological zones in both endemic and non-endemic areas in Ghana over a two-year period that covered both the rainy and dry seasons. At each site, temperature, relative humidity, precipitation, land cover (i.e. normalized difference vegetation index (NDVI)) and elevation data were obtained. Each mosquito was morphologically and molecularly identified to *An. gambiae* s.s. and to its molecular forms, and then dissected for *W. bancrofti* infections. *Wuchereria bancrofti* specimens from previous epidemiological studies at Gomoa were included in the study. Cytochrome C Oxidase subunit 1 (COI) DNA sequences of *W. bancrofti* and *An. gambiae* s.s. were sequenced and analysed to determine their genetic relationships. To better understand the effects of environmental factors on the diversity within the *An. gambiae* s.s, the spatial distribution of the *An. gambiae* M and S molecular forms and associated environmental factors were determined, along with their relationships with disease occurrence using both spatial cluster and multiple regression analyses.

# Results and discussions

A total of 10,274 mosquitoes were collected of which 6,150 (59.9%) were *An. gambiae* s.l and 1,494 (24.3%) were *An. gambiae* s.s. The distribution of the *An. gambiae* M and S forms varied significantly across the country and both occurred as sympatric populations at most locations. Spatial cluster analysis revealed a positive, spatial correlation of the *An. gambiae* M form (MI =0.19, Z score=4.2, $P<0.01$) and *An. gambiae* S form (MI =0.19, Z score=4.2, $P<0.01$) with their geographic location, which indicated that their distribution was influenced by distinct environmental factors and habitat characteristics. Multiple regression analysis revealed temperature as a key factor influencing the distribution of the two forms, and explained the dominance of the M form, 28% ($R^2=0.28$, F=25.8, P<0.001) in the savanna zones and the S form, 36% ($R^2=0.36$, F=37.9, P<0.001) in the middle forest belt. It was observed that the disease prevalence was significantly correlated with the occurrence of *An. gambiae* M being 2.5 to 3 times more abundant in the high LF transmission zone than in low-medium LF transmission zones (Fig.15. 1). The disease distribution in Ghana has the highest prevalence in the hotter Guinea/Sudan/Sahel savanna areas, which are also *An. gambiae* M form predominant areas. Phylogenetic analysis of the COI DNA sequences revealed two major clusters of south and north *W. bancrofti* populations (Fig. 15.2).

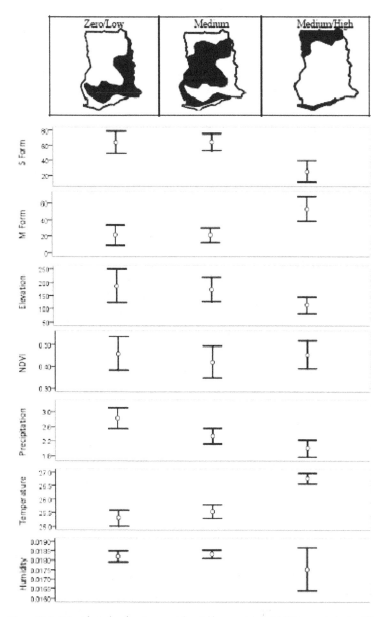

Figure 15.1: Entomological and environmental variables associated with LF transmission in different zones of Ghana. It shows that the An. gambiae s.s. M form and high temperatures were significantly associated with high LF transmission zone, and S form and lower temperatures with zero-medium transmission zones.

Hunter[14] and Ijumba and Lindsay[15] have both suggested that the Mopti form of *An. gambiae s.s.* are associated with *W. bancrofti* transmission. The distribution map of Gyapong *et al.*,[13] indicates that the incidence of the disease in West Africa is highest in the hotter Guinea/Sudan/Sahel savanna regions, which are also areas where the *An. gambiae* Mopti chromosomal form predominates.[16,17] Consequently, the existence of high LF prevalence in hotter areas of Ghana may be explained by the predominance of the *An. gambiae* M form. The genetic make-up of the vectors is thought to predispose them to defects, such as the absence of cibarial teeth.[18,19] For example, *Aedes* species exhibit the phenomenon of "limitation",[20] due to the absence of cibarial teeth.[18,21] Studies undertaken in the Gomoa District of Ghana found the number of cibarial teeth to differ significantly between the *An. gambiae* s.s. M and S forms with the M form having less number of teeth.[11] Thus, a smaller number of teeth means more parasites could pass through with less damage, and this could explain the high prevalence of LF in *An. gambiae* M form-dominant areas.

Our studies also found evidence of significant differences between *W. bancrofti* populations in the north and south of Ghana. It has been hypothesized that W. bancrofti was dispersed from Southeast Asia to Africa around 3,000 years ago by infected seafarers,[22] probably reaching Ghana and other Western African countries. Our results showed that the parasites in the south could have been the progenitors of those in the north (Fig 15.2) and also provide relevant information about the possible route of entry of *W. bancrofti* into Ghana and its subsequent spread. As observed for the forest and savanna forms of *Onchocerca volvulus*,[23] which respectively cause the non-blinding and blinding forms of onchocerciasis, the geographic strains of parasites may be important in disease pathogenicity. The observed genetic differences in the northern and southern populations of *W. bancrofti* could explain the higher prevalence of LF symptoms observed in the north compared to the south (Fig.15.2), but this requires further studies. Secondly, the difference observed in the LF epidemiology may be manifested in differences in virulence and pathogenicity of *W. bancrofti* infections observed in the north and south of Ghana.[24] In fact, suboptimal treatment responses in *W. bancrofti*[25] and selection for benzimidazole resistance in northern Ghana and Burkina Faso have also been reported.[26] However, before definitive conclusions could be made, further studies need to be done.

In conclusion, environmental factors, especially temperature, play an important role in the distribution of LF and its vectors in Ghana. Higher temperatures were preferred by *An. gambiae* ss. M form which in turn coincides with areas of high LF prevalence. The preponderance of the *An. gambiae* s.s. M form in the middle belt suggest that the S form is a benign vector. The cluster analysis grouped the southern *W. bancrofti* populations together, and from the phylogenetic branching, the south could have been the source of the ancestor population that spread to the north.

## 2  Identification of *Mansonia* species as vectors of lymphatic filariasis in Ghana

### Introduction

Various studies have always identified the *Anopheles gambiae* s.l. and *An. funestus* group as the only vectors of LF in Ghana. Although a previous report from Guinea[27] had incriminated *Mansonia* species as vectors in Guinea in the 1950s it had not been considered by researchers as meriting study in Ghana. Results obtained after seven rounds of annual mass drug administration (MDA) indicated that there were still sustained low levels of transmission in some areas where *An. melas*, *An. gambiae* s.s., *Mansonia* and *Culex* species occur in sympatry. Since *An. gambiae* s.l. and *An. funestus* are the known vectors there was a need to investigate whether any of the other mosquito-biting species could also be playing a role in the continued transmission of LF. We have earlier shown that the *Culex* species are not vectors[7] so we studied the *Mansonia* species.

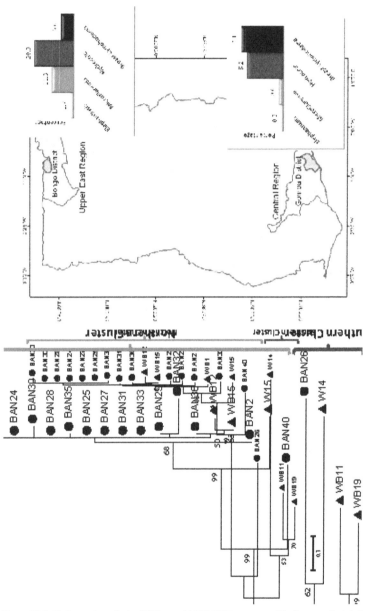

*Figure 15.2: Phylogenetic analysis of W. bancrofti COI DNA sequences: The figure on the left shows the phylogenetic tree obtained which reveals two clusters of north and south W. bancrofti. The map on the right shows the sites of collection and the charts (source: Gyapong et al.[24]) reveals differences in the prevalence of LF symptoms in the two areas.*

## Approach

Mosquitoes were collected indoors over a three-month period using pyrethrum spray catches in six communities within the Komenda-Edina-Eguafo-Abirem (KEEA) District, Ghana. The *Mansonia* species were identified morphologically and then dissected under a microscope, for *W. bancrofti* infections. *Mansonia* species obtained by a previous study conducted in the Gomoa District were similarly treated. The polymerase chain reaction method was used to confirm the identities of all the obtained *W. bancrofti* parasites.

## Findings and discussions

A total of 239 indoor resting *Mansonia* species were obtained and were dissected for the presence of *W. bancrofti*. Five hundred and one *An. gambiae* s.l. were similarly processed. The *Mansonia* species identified were *M. africana* and *M. uniformis* and the infection and infectivity rates were 2.5% and 2.1% respectively. *Anopheles gambiae* s.l. had infection and infectivity rates of 0.4%. From the stored mosquitoes, the infection and infectivity rates for *M. africana* were 7.6% (N=144) and 2.8% respectively whilst the corresponding rates for *M. uniformis* were 2.9% (N=244) and 0.8%.

This is the first report of *Mansonia* species as vectors of LF in Ghana. This previously unrecognised vector, which is probably more efficient than the known vectors, requires further studies to determine if they exhibit limitation. Should that be the case, then vector control should be added to mass drug adminitration (MDA) to achieve elimination of lymphatic filariasis in Ghana.

# 3 Impact of future climate change and control of nuisance bites of onchocerciasis vectors *Simulium damnosum* s.l. in the Volta basin, Ghana

## Introduction

Onchocerciasis (river blindness) as its common name suggests is associated with rivers and streams. It is a debilitating disease infecting approximately 37,000,000 people globally of whom about 500,000 are blind and 1,000,000 visually impaired.[28] The disease is endemic in 30 sub-Saharan African countries and the estimated burden of disease in terms of disability-adjusted life years (DALYs) is 494,000 for 2010.[29] The disease is caused by a nematode worm *Onchocerca volvulus* and is transmitted in West Africa by blackflies of the *S. damnosum* species complex. The members of this complex differ in their ecologies and ability to transmit the disease. There are also differences in the severity of the disease according to bioclimatic zones, with savanna-dwelling taxa being the most efficient vectors associated with the severe disease.

The Intergovernmental Panel on Climate Change (IPCC) has shown that climate change contributes to the maintenance or otherwise of human health.[30] The IPCC estimates that some parts of Africa will become warmer and wetter whereas others become drier, and there will be changes in the frequencies of storms and floods. In future, the climate in endemic areas will either exacerbate the negative effects of onchocerciasis and fly bites, or will ameliorate conditions depending on whether it will either be hotter and wetter or cooler and drier because of the disease's association with rivers (i.e. discharges) and the biology of the *Simulium* vectors (i.e. developmental rates).

There is still no cure for onchocerciasis, therefore, changes in the geographical distribution and the severity of the disease is to be expected in response to environmental change, particularly climate-induced changes. As recognized by the Millennium Ecosystem Assessment,[31] deforestation has led to changes in the distribution of savanna members of the *S. damnosum* complex in Liberia[32] and Ghana.[33] Drier climatic regions would lead to savanna replacing forest species. Also, wetter climates would cause increased river discharge rates.

Obuobie *et al.* (unpublished data) predicted that rainfall would increase by 2.3% and ambient temperature by 3°C by 2100. Based on these information, Cheke (unpublished data) predicted that these would lead to 0.2% – 3.8% increases in fly numbers, depending on the season, culminating in about 3,000 more flies per annum at Asubende (R. Pru,) a community in the Black Volta basin. Cheke (unpublished data) also predicted that a projected increase in ambient temperatures by 2100 would lead to a 1°C increase in water temperatures which is likely to lead to the displacement of the comparatively benign vector *S. squamosum* by the efficient vector *S. damnosum* in the Volta basin by the end of this century or earlier. The implications are that onchocerciasis transmission will become more intense at sites where it is still occurring.

Inhabitants of onchocerciasis-endemic communities suffer from two key issues, both with negative health and socioeconomic impacts: the disease symptoms that ultimately result in blindness and severe skin lesions, and the biting nuisance of *Simulium* vectors which disturbs people and ultimately, reduces their productivity. Studies conducted in communities in the Black Volta basin found the majority of inhabitants declaring that the most immediate concern of onchocerciasis was the nuisance bites of blackflies (Osei-Akoto, unpublished data). One respondent in the study commented *The black flies come in their numbers and when you are weeding and you are not careful, you will cut your leg with your cutlass. I hate these organisms! If they were men like me, I would have engaged them in fierce battle!!* (Osei-Akoto, unpublished data). A case in point that emphasizes the gravity of the bites of blackflies was in 2009, when workers and residents threatened to vacate the Bui Dam site because of the intolerable nuisance which nearly led to the suspension of construction activities (http://www.modernghana.com/news/240480/1/black-flies-invade-bui-again.html)

Although studies have used plant materials to investigate protection against fly bites,[34,35,36] their feasibility for large-scale application remains in doubt because of the limited availability of the plant source. We therefore decided to investigate the effectiveness of commercially available insect repellents as better alternatives to control nuisance bites, especially, in view of the projected worsening onchocerciasis situation in the Volta basin.

## Approach

Five *N, N* -diethyl-3-methylbenzamide (DEET) products with active concentrations of 9.3%, 13%, 25%, 50% and 98.1-100% and a non-DEET product (active components: para-menthane-3, 8-diol and lemon grass oil) were purchased and tested at Bui-Agblekame, Ghana. Eight groups comprising two vector collectors each used either repellents (treatment, or mineral oil) or nothing each day on rotational basis until the end of the study. The repellents were applied on the legs before fly catches commenced at 07.00 am. Flies were caught and their numbers for each hour recorded using the standard methods for blackfly transmission studies.[37] The biting pressure i.e. mean daily biting rate (number of flies/person/day) was estimated and the percentage protection of each repellent calculated using the equation: percentage protection = $[(T - C)/C] \times 100$ (where T = flies landing on treatments and C = flies landing on controls). Two-way t-test comparisons between each set of repellents were done. Analysis of variance involving two factors (catchers and repellents) was also conducted, with total flies caught as the dependent variable, followed by Tukey's tests which compared the total numbers of flies caught for all the tested repellents. A p-value of less than 0.05 was considered to be statistically significant.

Following from the field experiments, the non-DEET product was selected and tested on 75 Bui Dam construction workers over five days to determine if twice daily applications (morning and midday) would provide complete protection. The workers were asked to respond to five questions after the trial:

1. Did two application of the repellent offered complete protection?
2. Did they liked the smell?
3. Were there any adverse side-effects?
4. Were they willing to use it all the time?
5. Were they willing to recommend it to employers?

## Results and Discussions

The highest percentage protection of 80.8% was achieved by the non-DEET product and the lowest of 42.5% by the 13% DEET product. The period of absolute protection was 5 hours by the non-DEET (range 5-7 hours) and 1hour by the 50% DEET product. Moreover, the waning of the non-DEET product was slower than that of the DEET-based repellents (Fig.15.3). It was then hypothesized that twice daily application of the non-DEET product might therefore offer complete protection during the day when flies are active. The field trial of the non-DEET repellent was conducted with 75 construction workers. Amongst them, 98.7% reported complete protection, 95.9% of 73 respondents liked the smell, 68% of 75 participants reported no adverse side-effects while 29% reported transient nausea, 98.6% and 98.7% respectively agreed to daily use and to recommend it to their employers.

# Conclusion

In the event of future climate change scenarios of warmer and wetter conditions, the relief from increased nuisance bites by the *S. damnosum* s.l. vectors could be achieved through the extensive use of the non-DEET repellent by inhabitants in endemic areas. These findings have generated further research which aims at investigating the cost-effectiveness, community user-acceptance, impact and feasibility of repellent use as an additional tool for onchocerciasis control in the Volta basin.

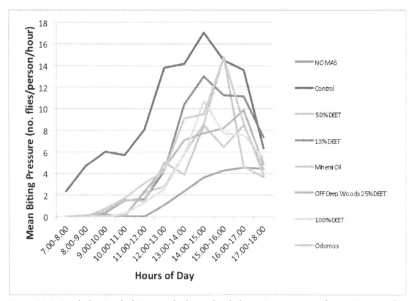

*Figure 15.3: Graph showing the biting trends observed with the various treatments from 7.00 am until the end of the period of catching (Source: Wilson et al. [38]).*

# Acknowledgments

We wish to acknowledge the immense contributions of Josephine Ughasi, Hilaria Esiawonam Bekard, Maimouna Coulibaly, Delphina Adabie-Gomez, John Gyapong and Maxwell Appawu of NMIMR, ,along with Isaac Osei-Akoto and George Domfe both of ISSER; Mike Osei-Atweneboana and Emmanuel Obuobie of Water Research Institute, CSIR; Anthony Kiszewski of Bentley University, USA; Robert A Cheke, University of Greenwich, UK and Carl Wiafe in generating some of the information contained in this article. Drs. Obuobie, Isaac Osei-Akoto and Robert Cheke granted us the permission to use their data. We acknowledge the support by DfID/IDRC Canada to MDW, WHO/TDR grant award to DAB, Gates Foundation grant and the African Regional Postgraduate Programme for Insect Scientists (ARPPIS) fellowship award to Josephine Ughasi are acknowledged.

# References

1.  World Health Organization. *Eliminating Lymphatic Filariasis*. Geneva: WHO, 2000.
2.  World Health Organization. *Annual Report of the Global Programme to Eliminate Lymphatic Filariasis*. Geneva: WHO, 2002.
3.  Dunyo, S. K., Appawu, M. A., Nkrumah, F. K. *et al.* Lymphatic filariasis on the coast of Ghana. *Trans Roy Soc Trop Med Hyg.*1996; 90: 634-638.
4.  Ahorlu, C. K., Dunyo, S. K., Koram, K. A. *et al.* Lymphatic filariasis related perceptions and practices on the coast of Ghana: implications for prevention and control. *Acta Tropica.* 1999; 73: 251-264.
5.  Dzodzomenyo, M. D., Dunyo, S. K., Ahorlu, C. K. *et al.* Bancroftian filariasis in an irrigation project community in southern Ghana. *Trop Med Int Health* 1999; 4:13-18.
6.  Appawu, M. A., Dadzie, S. K., Wilmot-Baffoe, A. *et al.* Lymphatic filariasis in Ghana: entomological investigation of transmission dynamics and intensity in communities served by irrigation systems in the Upper East Region of Ghana. *Trop Med Int Health.* 2001; 6:511-516.
7.  Aboagye-Antwi, F. Studies on the Roles of *Culex* and *Anopheles* species in the transmission of *Wuchereria bancrofti (Spirurida: Filariidae)* in

the Gomoa District of Ghana [Unpublished Dissertation]. Zoology Department: University of Ghana; 2003.

8.  Ughasi, J., Bekhard, H., Coulibaly, M. *et al. Mansonia africana* and *Mansonia uniformis* are vectors in the transmission of *Wuchereria bancrofti* lymphatic filariasis in Ghana. *Parasites and Vectors.* 2012; 5:89.

9.  Boakye, D. A., Wilson, M. D., Appawu, M. A. *et al.* Vector competence, for *Wuchereria bancrofti*, of the *Anopheles* populations in the Bongo district of Ghana. *Ann Trop Med Parasitol.* 2004; 98:501-508.

10. Clement, I. Vector competence of *Anopheles gambiae* s.l (*Diptera: Culicidae*) populations for *Wuchereria bancrofti* (*Spirurida: Filaridae*) at low microfilaraemia along the coast in the Western Region of Ghana. [Unpublished Dissertation]. Zoology Department: University of Ghana; 2006.

11. Amuzu, H., Wilson, M., Boakye, D. Studies of *Anopheles gambiae* s.l (Diptera: Culicidae) exhibiting different vectorial capacities in lymphatic filariasis transmission in the Gomoa District, Ghana. *Parasite and Vectors.* 2010; 3:85.

12. de Souza, D. K. Diversity in *Anopheles gambiae* s.s and *Wuchereria bancrofti*, and the Distribution of Lymphatic Filariasis in Ghana. [Unpublished Dissertation]. Department of Theoretical and Applied Biology: Kwame Nkrumah University of Science and Technology, 2010.

13. Gyapong, J. O., Kyelem, D., Kleinschmidt, I. *et al.* The use of spatial analysis in mapping the distribution of bancroftian filariasis in four West African countries. *Ann Trop Med Parasitol.* 2002; 96:695-705.

14. Hunter, J. M. Elephantiasis: a disease of development in north east Ghana. *Soc Sci Med.* 1992; 35:627-645.

15. Ijumba, J. N., Lindsay, S. W. Impact of irrigation on malaria in Africa: paddies paradox. *Med Vet Entomol.* 2001; 15:1-11.

16. Bayoh, M. N., Thomas, C. J., Lindsay, S. W.. Mapping distributions of chromosomal forms of *Anopheles gambiae* in West Africa using climate data. *Med Vet Entomol.* 2001; 15:267-274.

17. Kelly-Hope, L. A., Diggle, P. J., Rowlingson, B. S. *et al.* Negative spatial association between lymphatic filariasis and malaria in West Africa. *Trop Med Int Health.*2006; 11: 129-135.

18. McGreevy, P. B., Bryan, J. H., Oothuman, P. *et al.* The lethal effects of the cibarial and pharyngeal armatures of mosquitoes on microfilariae. *Trans Roy Soc Trop Med Hyg.*1978; 72:361-368.

19. Lowrie, J. R. C. Poor vector efficiency of *Culex quinquefasciatus* following infection with *Dirofilaria immitis. J Am Mosq Control Assoc.* 1991; 7:30-36.

20. Pichon, G. Limitation and facilitation in the vectors and other aspects of the dynamics of filarial transmission: the need for vector control against *Anopheles* transmitted filariasis. *Ann Trop Med Parasitol.* 2002; 96: S143-S152.

21. McGreevy, P. B., Kolstrup, N., Tao, J. *et al.* Ingestion and development of *Wuchereria bancrofti* in *Culex quinquefasciatus, Anopheles gambiae* and *Aedes aegypti* after feeding on humans with varying densities of microfilariae in Tanzania. *Trans Roy Soc Trop Med Hyg.* 1982; 76: 288-296.

22. Laurence, B.R. The global dispersal of bancroftian filariasis. *Parasitol Today.* 1989; 5: 260-265.

23. Zimmerman, P. A., Dadzie, K. Y., De Sole, G. E. R. *et al. Onchocerca volvulus* DNA probe classification correlates with epidemiologic patterns of blindness. *J Infect Dis.* 1992; 165: 964-968.

24. Gyapong, J., Adjei, S., Sackey, S. Descriptive epidemiology of lymphatic filariasis in Ghana. *Trans Roy Soc Trop Med Hyg.* 1996; 90: 26-30.

25. Eberhard, M. L., Lammie, P. L., Dickinson, C. M. *et al.* (1991) Evidence of non-susceptibility to diethylcarbamazine in *Wuchereria bancrofti. J Infect Dis.* 1991; 163: 1157-1160.

26. Schwab, A. E., Boakye, D. A., Kyelem, D., *et al.* Detection of benzimidazole resistance-associated mutations in the filarial nematode *Wuchereria bancrofti* and evidence for selection by Albendazole and Ivermectin combination treatment. *Am J Trop Med Hyg.* 2005; 73: 234-238.

27. Toumanoff, C. Filariose humaine et sa transmission dans la Basse-Guinée (Estuaire du Rio Nunez). *Bull Soc Pathol Exo.* 1958; 51: 908-912

28. Noma, M., Nwoke, B. E. B., Nutall, I. *et al.* Rapid epidemiological mapping of onchocerciasis (REMO): Its application by the African Programme for Onchocerciasis Control (APOC). *Ann Trop Med Parasitol.* 2002; 96: 29-39.

29. Murray, C. J. L., Vos, T., Lozano, R. *et al.* Disability-adjusted life years (DALYS) for 291 diseases and injuries in 21 Regions, 1990–2010: A systematic analysis for the global burden of disease study 2010. *Lancet.* 2012; 380: 2197-2223.

30. Intergovernmental Panel on Climate Change. Climate Change: The Physical Science Basis. Contribution of Working Group I to the Fourth Assessment Report of the Intergovernmental Panel on Climate Change (eds. Solomon S. *et al.*). 2007. Cambridge:Cambridge Univ. Press.

31. Millennium Ecosystem Assessment. Ecosystems and Human Well-being: Biodiversity Synthesis. 2005. Washington DC: World Resources Institute

32. Garms, R., Cheke, R. A., Sachs, R.. A. temporary focus of savanna species of the *Simulium damnosum* complex in the forest zone of Liberia. *Trop Med Parasitol.* 1991; 42: 181-187.

33. Wilson, M. D., Cheke, R. A., Flasse, S. P. J. *et al.* Deforestation and the spatio-temporal distribution of savanna and forest members of the *Simulium damnosum* complex in southern Ghana and south-western Togo. *Trans Roy Soc Trop Med Hyg.* 2002; 96: 632-639.

34. Opoku, A. K., Raybould, J. N., Kessie, D. K. Preliminary field evaluation of the repellent 'Simno' against the black fly *Simulium damnosums.l.*,a biting midge and mosquitoes. *Int J Trop Insect Sci.* 1986; 7: 31-36.

35. Pitroipa, X., Sankara, D., Konan, L. *et al.* Evaluation of cocoaoil for individual protection against *Simulium damnosum* s.l. *Medicine Tropicale: Revuedu Corps de Sante' Colonial.* 2002; 62: 511-516.

36. Sylla, M., Konan, L., Doannio, J. M. *et al.* Evaluation of the efficacy of coconut (*Cocos nucifera*), palm nut (*Eleadis guineensis*) and gobi (*Carapa procera*) lotions and creams in individual protection against *Simulium damnosum* s.l. in Côte d'Ivoire. *B Soc Path Ex.* 2003; 96:104-109.

37. Walsh, J. F., Davies, J. B., Le Berre, R. *et al.* Standardization of criteria for assessing the effect of *Simulium* control in onchocerciasis control programmes. *Trans Roy Soc Trop Med Hyg.* 1978; 72(6): 675-676.

38. Wilson, M. D., Osei-Atweneboana, M., Boakye, D. A. *et al.* Efficacy of DEET and non-DEET-based insect repellents against bites of *Simulium damnosum* vectors of onchocerciasis. *Med Vet Entomol.* 2012; doi: 10.1111/j.1365-2915. 2012.01054.x

# Chapter 16
# Towards sustainable control of schistosomiasis and soil-transmitted helminthiasis: Deworming and education at Ada-Foah, Ghana

*Kwabena M. Bosompem, William K. Anyan Daniel Boamah,*
*Stephanie K. Adjovu, Irene Ayi, Joseph Quartey, Joshua*
*Adjovu, Jonas Asigbee, Maxwell A., Michael D. Wilson,*
*Daniel A. Boakye, Koichi Morinaka, Hisayoshi Ogiwara,*
*Nobuo Ohta and Tsutomu Takeuchi*

## Introduction

It is generally accepted that parasitic diseases are endemic in many developing countries and pose as obstacles to healthy growth and socio-economic development.[1] Infections caused by soil-transmitted helminthes (STH) and schistosomes are among the most prevalent parasitic afflictions of humans living in areas of poverty in the developing world with poor hygiene and sanitation.[2-5] An estimated 1.2 billion of the world's population is chronically infected with these STH (*Ascaris lumbricoides, Trichuris trichiura, Ancylostoma duodenale* and *Necatar americanus*) and schistosomes (*Schistosoma haematobium, S. mansoni* and *S. japonicum*),[6] and are responsible for growth retardation, anaemia and reduced learning ability in children as well as increased susceptibility to other infections.[7,8]

In recognition of the huge burden of parasitic diseases on health and socio-economic development in the world, the West African Centre for International Parasite Control (WACIPAC) was established with Japanese government support at the Noguchi Memorial Institute for Medical Research (NMIMR), as one of three Centres for International

Parasite Control (CIPACs) in Asia and Africa. Using the school-based approach, WACIPAC initiated treatment and education intervention for schistosomiasis and STH in its model project site.

# Approach

The study was conducted in Ada-Foah sub-district of the Dangme East District, Greater Accra Region, the WACIPAC model project site in Ghana. Ada-Foah, lies along the south-eastern coast of Ghana approximately 100 km east of the capital city, Accra at the River Volta estuary. The relief is generally flat with coastal savannah vegetation consisting mainly of grasses with isolated shrubs and trees. The climate is mostly dry during most parts of the year, with a mean annual rainfall ranging between 740-900mm. The highest and lowest mean monthly temperatures are about 30°C and 26°C respectively. The relative humidity, which is high throughout the year, ranges between 65-80%. Water contact points along tributaries of the River Volta and ponds serve as sources of fresh water for some inhabitants. The major occupations are fishing and salt mining. Ten (10) primary schools served the educational needs of school aged children in the sub-district.

Following approval and ethical clearance from the Scientific and Technical Committee, and the Institutional Review Board of NMIMR, permission was obtained from the Dangme East District Assembly as well as the District offices of the Ghana Education Service and the Ghana Health Service. Consent was also sought from community leaders, teachers and parents. Data on STH and schistosomiasis-related to knowledge, attitudes and practices (KAP) was collected using questionnaire interviews. Furthermore, parasitological data (obtained through microscopic analysis of stool and urine samples) was used to determine the prevalence, distribution and intensity of STH and schistosomiasis from baseline survey in 2002, and follow-ups in 2007 and 2008. In line with WHO guidelines for evaluation of school-based deworming programmes, pupils in class three were surveyed in each school.[9] The intervention programme involved treatment of infections, health education, and hygiene and sanitation promotion utilizing IEC materials developed by WACIPAC for behaviour change.

# Findings

As shown in Table 16.1, a total of 512 pupils were surveyed at baseline in 2002 as against 518 at follow-up in 2007 and 573 in 2008. In all surveys the male population was higher than the females; 923 males (57.6%) and 680 females (42.4%) (p > 0.05). In each survey, all pupils studied responded to the questionnaire, but not all provided stool and urine samples for parasitological analysis (Table 16.2). The ages ranged from 6 – 25 years.

Table 16.1    Showing the general characteristics of the study population.

| *Name of School | 2002 | | | | 2007 | |
|---|---|---|---|---|---|---|
| | Number involved | Male | Female | Age Range (years) | Number involved | Male |
| AFD | 39 | 22 | 17 | 8 - 24 | 58 | 32 |
| ANY | 67 | 41 | 26 | 8 - 18 | 50 | 37 |
| PUT | 96 | 65 | 31 | 7 - 16 | 51 | 23 |
| AFRC | 37 | 23 | 14 | 10 - 15 | 51 | 28 |
| AFM | 48 | 28 | 20 | 7 - 16 | 53 | 29 |
| AZI | 42 | 24 | 18 | 8 - 19 | 58 | 29 |
| ELA | 42 | 27 | 15 | 10 - 20 | 51 | 40 |
| OCN | 59 | 31 | 28 | 8 - 19 | 50 | 30 |
| TMK | 34 | 25 | 9 | 8 - 16 | 46 | 21 |
| AFP | 48 | 26 | 22 | 7 - 20 | 50 | 28 |
| Total | 512(100%) | 312(60.9%) | 200(39.1%) | 7 - 24 | 518(100%) | 297(57 |

* Name of School

| | | |
|---|---|---|
| AFD | - | Ada-Foah DA Primary |
| ANY | - | Anyakpor RC Primary |
| PUT | - | Pute Presbyterian 1 & 2 Primary |
| AFRC | - | Ada-Foah RC Primary |
| AFM | - | Ada-Foah Methodist Primary |
| AZI | - | Azizanya DA Primary |
| ELA | - | Elavanyo DC Primary |
| OCN | - | Ocanseykope DA Primary |
| TMK | - | Totimekope DA Primary |
| AFP | - | Ada-Foah Presbyterian Primary |

| Female | Age Range (years) | 2008 | | | |
| | | Number involved | Male | Female | Age Range (years) |
| --- | --- | --- | --- | --- | --- |
| 26 | 8 - 25 | 64 | 32 | 32 | 6 - 20 |
| 13 | 8 - 18 | 52 | 33 | 19 | 7 - 18 |
| 28 | 8 - 20 | 69 | 36 | 33 | 8 - 17 |
| 23 | 7 - 15 | 60 | 30 | 30 | 8 - 18 |
| 24 | 7 - 19 | 52 | 23 | 29 | 6 - 15 |
| 29 | 8 - 25 | 71 | 37 | 34 | 8 - 19 |
| 11 | 9 - 18 | 50 | 37 | 13 | 9 - 20 |
| 20 | 7 - 17 | 51 | 36 | 15 | 7 - 17 |
| 25 | 8 - 17 | 53 | 28 | 25 | 7 - 19 |
| 22 | 7 - 16 | 51 | 22 | 29 | 8 - 19 |
| 221(42.7%) | 7 - 25 | 573(100%) | 314(54.8%) | 259(45.2%) | 6 - 20 |

Table 16.2:  Distribution of questionnaires, urine and stool samples by
schools

| Name of School | 2002 | | | |
|---|---|---|---|---|
| | Number. of questionnaire analysed | Number. of Urine Samples | Number. of Stool Samples | Number. of questionnaire analysed |
| AFD | 39 | 37 | 36 | 58 |
| ANY | 67 | 62 | 62 | 50 |
| PUT | 96 | 93 | 93 | 51 |
| AFRC | 37 | 35 | 34 | 51 |
| AFM | 48 | 48 | 43 | 53 |
| AZI | 42 | 36 | 38 | 58 |
| ELA | 42 | 41 | 38 | 51 |
| OCN | 59 | 59 | 47 | 50 |
| TMK | 34 | 34 | 34 | 46 |
| AFP | 48 | 46 | 47 | 50 |
| Overall Total | 512(100%) | 491(95.9%) | 472(92.2%) | 518(100%) |

# Knowledge Attitudes and Practices

The pupils surveyed had access to seven different sources of water
namely, stream, pond, well, pipe-borne water, spring, rain water and
water tanks. The rate of utilization of the different sources of water
by the pupils differed at baseline and follow-up surveys. Well water
was the most frequently used; 72.2% at baseline, 79.0% at follow-up
in 2007 and 79.8% in 2008. This was followed by pipe-borne water;
39.0% at 2002, 37.2% in 2007 and 52.8% in 2008. The use of stream
water was highest at baseline; 19.9%, but this reduced to 8.5% in
2007 and then rose again to 16.3% in 2008. Rain water utilization
was 16.3% in 2007 and 5.2% in 2008. None of the pupils used rain
water in 2002. The least utilized source of water was the spring; 0.7%
in 2002, 0.7% in 2007 and none in 2008.

The survey revealed practices that influenced the transmission
of schistosomiasis. Approximately 40.0% of the pupils swam in the
river in 2007 and this increased to 49.1% in 2008 (p > 0.05). On the
other hand, 13.8% of the children avoided swimming in the river in

| 007 | | | 2008 | |
| --- | --- | --- | --- | --- |
| Number. of Urine amples | Number. of Stool Samples | Number. of questionnaire analysed | Number. of Urine Samples | Number. of Stool Samples |
| ·0 | 50 | 64 | 57 | 53 |
| ·9 | 50 | 52 | 46 | 42 |
| ·0 | 26 | 69 | 66 | 50 |
| ·5 | 35 | 60 | 57 | 55 |
| ·0 | 50 | 52 | 48 | 47 |
| ·7 | 48 | 71 | 55 | 53 |
| ·7 | 51 | 50 | 47 | 42 |
| ·5 | 49 | 51 | 49 | 49 |
| ·2 | 43 | 53 | 47 | 42 |
| ·7 | 49 | 51 | 50 | 49 |
| ·72(91.1%) | 451(87.1%) | 573(100%) | 522(91.1%) | 482(84.1%) |

2007 and this reduced to 11.5% in 2008. The percentage of children who urinated in or near the river or pond increased from 39.4% in 2007 to 49.1% in 2008. However, the percentage of children who do not urinate into water reduced from 4.8% in 2007 to 1.8% in 2008. Interestingly, the rate of defecation in or near the river or pond increased from 15.4% in 2007 to 19.6% in 2008 (p > 0.05).

Figure 16.1 shows practices that influence STH transmission among the school pupils. Majority of the children indicated that they ate with their hands; 99.8% in 2007 and 98.2% in 2008. However, fewer children washed hands before eating; 13.5% in 2007 and 6.9% in 2008. Furthermore, very few children washed hands after toilet; 9.6% in 2007 and only 0.3% in 2008. Interestingly, of those who washed their hands, a high percentage washed with soap; 80.3% in 2007 and 80.2 in 2008. The survey revealed that most of the children had shoes; 97.7% in 2007 and 98.3 in 2008 and most children wore their shoes to school. Fewer children indicated that they were dewormed regularly at home: 22.0% in 2007 and 24.2% in 2008.

A high percentage of pupils, 82.7% correctly indicated blood in urine as a sign/symptom of urinary schistosomiasis at baseline in 2002, compared to 21.0% in 2007 and 27.6% in 2008. Very few pupils (< 2.0%) identified malnutrition, anaemia and protruded abdomen as schistosomiasis signs/symptoms. Unlike urinary schistosomiasis, a lower percentage of pupils correctly indicating blood in stool as a sign/symptom of intestinal schistosomiasis; 17.1% in 2002, 3.1% in 2007 and 4.05% in 2008.

Throughout the study, pupils indicated "abdominal pains" as the main sign/symptom of STH; 24.7% in 2002, 19.5% in 2007 and 18.9% in 2008. Fewer children (< 5.0%) indicated malnutrition and anaemia as signs/symptoms of STH.

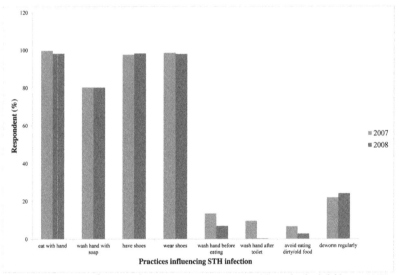

*Figure 16.1: Practices influencing schistosome transmission among Ada-Foah school children in 2007 and 2008.*

# Parasitological survey

Examination of urine and stool in the baseline survey revealed six (6) different parasites (*S. haematobium, S. mansoni, Ascaris sp., T. trichiura, H. nana* and Hookworms) that infected the school children.

As shown in Figure 16.2, there was a decline in the prevalence of *S. haematobium,* 11.2% in 2002 to 3.7% in 2007 and *S. mansoni,* 5.3% in 2002 to 2.2% in 2007. However, the prevalence of both infections increased in 2008; 11.7% for S. *haematobium* and 7.45% for S. *mansoni*. In the case of STH, there was a systematic reduction in the cumulative prevalence of (A. *lumbricoides*, T. *trichiura* and hookworms) from baseline 24.8% to 4.8% in 2008. The prevalence of A. *lumbricoides* infection showed a similar decline over the years, whilst hookworm infection was not detected in the final survey in 2008 (Figure 16.3). Generally there was a decline in prevalence of T. *trichiura* infection from 11.8% in 2002 to 1.1% in 2007, followed by a slight increase to 1.85% in 2008 ($p < 0.05$).

The intensity variation of urinary and intestinal schistosomiasis followed a similar pattern as the prevalence of infection (Figure 16.3). At baseline, the percentage of heavy intensity S. *haematobium* infection 5.6% was higher than the low intensity infections 3.9%. However, in the follow-up surveys in 2007 and 2008, the percentage of heavy intensity infections were lower than the light intensity infections (Figure 16.4). Generally, the intensity of S. *mansoni* infection followed a similar pattern with declining rates of moderate and heavy intensity infections over the years. Also, as illustrated in Figure 16.5, for A. *lumbricoides*, a similar trend of decreasing intensity variation was observed for T. *trichiura* and hookworm.

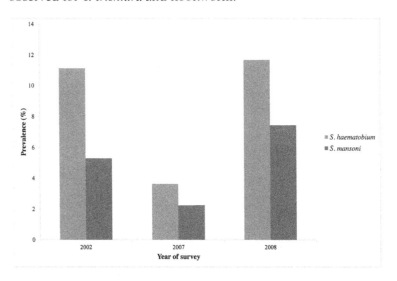

*Figure 16.2: Prevalence of S. haematobium and S. mansoni in Ada-Foah schools in 2002, 2007 and 2008.*

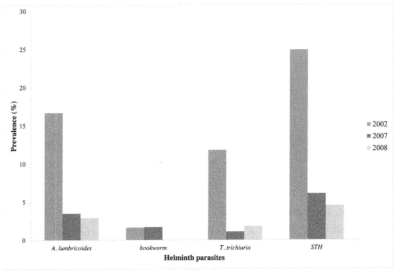

Figure 16.3: Prevalence of helminth infections in Ada-Foah school children in 2002, 2007 and 2008.

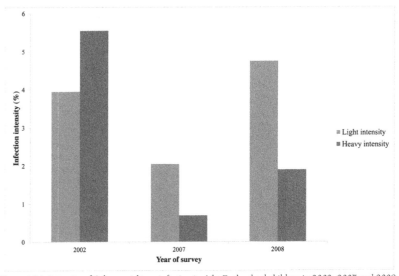

Figure 16.4: Intensity of S. haematobium infection in Ada-Foah school children in 2002, 2007 and 2008.

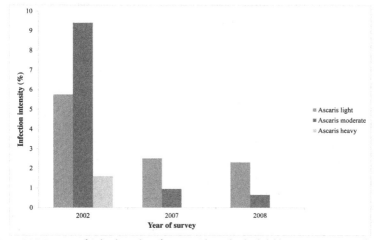

*Figure 16.5: Intensity of A. lumbricoides infection in Ada-Foah school children in 2002, 2007 and 2008.*

# Discussion

The aim of the study was to determine the status of schistosomiasis and STH in the WACIPAC model project site, Ada-Foah sub-district, following school-based parasitic diseases intervention activities. The study was conducted in all 10 basic schools at the project site.

The use of school-based health promoting activities for the control of schistosomiasis and STH among school-age children by the WACIPAC is a preferred option in developing countries.[10] This is because children present the highest intensity of worm infection, which impacts negatively on all aspects of their health, nutrition, cognitive development, learning, and access to education and academic achievement.[7,8,11,12]

Montresor and others[3] reported that in order to obtain comparable data from different control programmes, pupils in third year primary school (Class 3), should be surveyed. In this study, pupils in primary three were surveyed following the recommendations of WHO Expert Committee on Deworming.[12] The number of school children (512 pupils) surveyed in the baseline in 2002 was comparable to the numbers involved in the follow-up years, 518 in 2007and 573 in 2008 (p > 0.05).[13]

The reported defecation and urination along the banks of water bodies in the communities despite deworming and health education activities, highlighted challenges with maintaining positive behaviour change among the pupils. This habit of contamination of rivers and ponds with human urine and stool from individuals infected with schistosomiasis introduces schistosome ova that promotes transmission of the disease.[14] Bruun and Aagaard-Hansen,[14] pointed out that increased transmission of schistosomiasis exposes children and other community folks to the infections. This may partly explain the increased prevalence of schistosomiasis at the end of the study in 2008. It may also explain the observed high proportion of pupils with heavy infections of both *S. haematobium* and *S. mansoni*. Finally, the continuous engagement of pupils in swimming reported in this study maintains their contact with schistosome infested rivers and ponds.

Sama and Ratard[19] and Wagatsuma and colleagues[16] found an association between prior infection of individuals and their higher levels of knowledge about the infection. Similarly, in this research, a higher proportion of pupils who indicated they knew of STH had suffered from the disease. Although health education was continued after baseline survey, the percentage of pupils who considered not swimming in the river as the best way of controlling schistosomiasis was higher at baseline in 2002. This percentage however decreased significantly in the schools in 2007 and 2008 probably accounting for the observed increase in the number of pupils who swim in rivers/ponds.

Proper personal hygiene and environmental sanitation in addition to regular deworming are essential for the control of STH.[19] These include the washing of hands with soap before eating and after visiting the toilet, and wearing of shoes. Even though high proportion of pupils who ate with their hands, did not wash their hands before eating and after toilet, the prevalence of STH declined consistently. This observation may be partly explained by the inclusion of regular deworming in the control activities. The use of soap by a high percentage of the children who washed their hands before eating is also a likely contributing factor. In addition, the observation that a large proportion of pupils in this study had shoes and they wore them, may explain the apparent disappearance of hookworm infections by 2008. Ultimately the health education component of the school-based health promotion activities employed in the WACIPAC intervention programme appears to have positively impacted on personal hygiene and led to a reduction in the prevalence of STH. A similar observation was made by Kobayashi and colleagues[17] in which the prevalence rates of the major STH infections declined in the model schools of the Asian Center of International Parasite Control (ACIPAC) involved in health promoting school activities.

The fluctuating changes in the prevalence of urinary and intestinal schistosomiasis over the years: 2002 through 2007 to 2008 is plausible as has been demonstrated in control programs in Kenya and elsewhere.[18]

Heavy intensity of infections,[19] with *T. trichiura* were reported in the baseline survey in 2002 but not in 2007 and 2008. The absence of heavy intensity infection with *T. trichiura* and *A. lumbricoides* after the baseline survey in 2002 shows that the intervention measures had a positive influence in reducing the prevalence of this infection.

Generally, from this study it can be observed that parasitological intervention activities of WACIPAC have had a positive influence in reducing the prevalence and intensities of STH, as well as the intensities of schistosomiasis in the Ada-Foah Sub District of the Dangme East district. There was however limited knowledge of the causes, signs and symptoms, and the best ways to control schistosomiasis and STH. Such knowledge gaps could limit systematic reduction of the infections to the point of elimination or eradication in the study schools. These knowledge gaps may be partly attributed to regular turnover of pupils in the schools as well as replacement of teachers through transfers. There is therefore the need to focus more on monitoring and evaluation of intervention strategies employed by WACIPAC so as to effectively interrupt the transmission of schistosomiasis and STH and to bring about sustainable improvement in the knowledge and behaviour of school pupils towards the control of these diseases.

# Acknowledgements

We gratefully acknowledge Mr. O. Agyeman-Duah, Mr. R. A. Appai, Mr. Samuel Mortu, Mr. Isaac Adjaottor, Mr. Felix Yorhu, Mr. David Glover and Ms. D. Joppa for technical assistance. We are also thankful to Dr. S. Yamaguchi, Prof. S. Kojima, Dr. John Yabani, Dr. R. Y. Osei, Mrs Mary Quaye, Mrs. Vida Drapson and Mr. Kofi Plahar for the invaluable assistance in conducting this work and Messrs Francis Anan, Joseph

Asare and Stephen Otoo for driving our research team to the field. We are also grateful to the Ada-Foah community members and school teachers for their support of the intervention activities. This research was undertaken with joint financial assistance from the Government of Ghana and the Japan International Cooperation Agency (JICA).

# References

1.  WHO. *Bench Aids for the Diagnosis of Intestinal Parasites*. World Health Organisation, Geneva. (1994).

2.  Giles, H.M. Soil-Transmitted Helminths (Geohelminths). In Cook, G., ed. (20th ed., 1996). *Manson's Tropical Disease*. WB Saunders, London.

3.  Montresor, A., Crompton, D. W. T., Hall, A., Bundy, D. A. P., and Savioli, L: *Guidelines for the Evaluation of Soil-Transmitted Heliminthiasis and Schistosomiasis at community level*. WHO, Geneva. (1998).

4.  Hotez, P., J., Brindley, P. J., Bethony, J. M., King, C. H., Pearce, E. J. and Jacobson, J. Helminth Infections: The Great Neglected Tropical Diseases. *J Clin Invest*. (2008) 118(4): 1311–1321. doi: 10.1172/JCI34261.

5.  WHO: *Working to overcome the global impact of neglected tropical diseases: first WHO report on neglected tropical diseases*: World Health Organization; 2010.http//:whqlibdoc.who.int/publications/2010/9789241564090_eng.pdf.

6.  Hotez, P. J., Fenwick, A., Savioli, L., Molyneux D. H. Rescuing the "bottom billion" through neglected tropical disease control. *Lancet* 2009, 373:1570–1576.

7.  Stephenson, L. S. *Impact of Helminth Infections on Human Nutrition*. Taylor and Francis, London; (1987). 50.

8.  Stephenson, L. S, Crompton, D.W. T., Latham, M. C., Schulpen, T. W. I., Nesheim, M. C and Jansen, A. A. G. Relationship between *Ascaris* Infection and Growth of Malnourished Pre-school children in Kenya. *Am J Clin Nutr*; (1980). 33: 1165-1172.

9.  Montresor, A., Crompton, D. W. T, Hall, A., Bundy, D. A. P, Savioli, L. Guidelines for the Evaluation of Soil-transmitted Helminthiasis and Schistosomiasis at Community Level. A Guide for Managers of Control Programmes, WHO/CTD/SIP/98.1, Geneva. (1998), 1-45.

10. Hotez, P. J., Bundy, D. A. P, Beegle, K, Brooker, S, Drake, L, de Silva, N, Montresor, A., Engels, D., Jukes, M., Chitsulo, L., Chow, J.,

Correa-Oliveira, R., Shu-Hua, X., Fenwick, A. and Savioli, L. Helminth Infections: Soil-transmitted Helminth Infections and Schistosomiasis. In: *Disease control priorities in developing countries*. 2nd ed., edited by Dean T. Jamison, Joel G. Breman, Anthony R. Measham, George Alleyne, Mariam Claeson *et al.*, Washington, D.C., World Bank. (2006), 467-482.

11. World Bank. School Deworming at a Glance. *Public Health at a Glance Series*. www.worldbank.org. (2003).

12. WHO (2003). School Deworming at a Glance. *WHO Technical Report Series*, Geneva. (2003). 912

13. GCPI Secretariat. *Global Parasite Control Initiative in West Africa: Baseline Surveys for Parasitic Diseases in the Ada-Foah Sub District, Dangme East District, Ghana (November-December, 2002) Report*. The Secretariat, Noguchi Memorial Institute for Medical Research, Legon, Ghana. (2003).

14. Bruun, B., and Aagaard-Hansen, J. The social context of schistosomiasis and its control: an introduction and annotated bibliography. Switzerland: World Health Organization. (2008) 213 p.

15. Sama, M. T and Ratard, R. C. Water Contact and Schistosomiasis Infection in Kumba, South-Western Cameroon. *Annals of Tropical Medicine and Parasiotology*. (1994). 88(6):629-634.

16. Wagatsuma, Y., Aryeetey, M. E., Nkrumah, F. K., Sack, D. A. and Kojima, S. Highly Symptom-Aware Children were Heavily Infected with Urinary Schistosomiasis in Southern Ghana. *Cent Afr J of Med*, (2003). 49:16-19

17. Kobayashi, J., Socheat, D., Phommasack, B., Tun, A., and Nga, N. H. Activities in Partner Countries (Cambodia, Lao PDR, Myanmar and Vietnam): Small Scale Pilot Project (SSPP) and Other Impacts. The Asian Center of International Parasite Control (ACIPAC): Five Years of Achievement. The *Southeast Asian J of Trop Med Public Health*, (2005) 36 (3): 28-37.

18. King, C. H. Longterm Outcomes of School-Based Treatment for Control of Urinary Schistosomiasis: A Review of Experience in Coast Province, Kenya. *Mem Inst Oswaldo Cruz*, Rio de Janeiro, (2006) 101 (1):299-306.

19. Montresor, A., Crompton, D. W. T., Gyorkos, T. W. and Savioli, L. *Helminth Control in School-Age Children: A Guide for Managers of Control Programmes*. WHO, Geneva. (2002).

# Chapter 17
# Investigations to support the prevention and management of HIV in Ghana

*William K. Ampofo and Evelyn Yayra Bonney*

## Introduction

The human immunodeficiency virus (HIV) epidemic in Ghana is described as 'generalized' with a low national HIV prevalence of 1.37% in 2012.[1] In 1986, when the first HIV/AIDS was identified in Ghana, a total of 42 cases were reported.[2] Recent estimates indicated that 235,982 people were living with HIV in Ghana and 7,991 persons were newly infected in 2012.[1] The 2012 HIV sentinel survey report indicated that both HIV-1 and HIV-2 co-circulate in Ghana with HIV-1 being the predominant type with 96.4% followed by 2.9% for HIV-1/2 dual infections and 0.7% for HIV-2.[3] However, the HIV-1 subtypes have evolved over the years from the era of dominance of pure A and G subtypes[4] to the era where circulating recombinant forms (CRFs) particularly CRF02_AG is the predominant HIV-1 subtype in Ghana.[5, 6, 7, 8.]

Genetic diversity of HIV has implications for viral fitness and replication, susceptibility to antiretroviral drugs and selection of specific drug resistance mutations under drug pressure.[9] The Noguchi Memorial Institute for Medical Research (NMIMR) has worked in areas such as laboratory confirmation of HIV antibodies in blood samples of persons with indeterminate results, external quality assurance for the HIV sentinel survey (HSS) samples, molecular probing to resolve the HIV status of persons exposed to needle-stick injuries during clinical care, babies born to HIV-infected mothers and the monitoring of drug resistance among patients on antiretroviral therapy. The NMIMR boasts of a high level of research expertise in the area of HIV and AIDS and the provision of important data to guide national intervention programmes. This treatise highlights two of such research: (1) A study to determine a factor – the false recent rate of HIV infection to guide the future application of assays to measure incidence of HIV infection in Ghana and (2) Serological profiling of HIV infected patients in Ghana, to highlight the important contribution of the Noguchi Memorial Institute for Medical Research to the national response in the prevention and management of HIV infections in Ghana.

# 1. Seroepidemiology: baseline study to enable measurement of HIV incidence

In Ghana, HIV prevalence in the general population is determined by the HIV sentinel surveys (HSS). These annual HIV sentinel surveys have been conducted among pregnant women aged 15 – 49 years at selected antenatal facilities since 1992. The survey is based on the premise that prevalence of HIV among pregnant women is a good proxy indicator of the spread of the infection among the populace[2]. The HSS has served as the principal database for National HIV and AIDS estimates.

In 2003, the Ghana Demographic and Health Survey (GDHS) included for the first time, blood collection for HIV testing. The NMIMR was responsible for the conduct of this biomarker investigation which generated a reference indicator enabling the application of the Estimation Projection Package for HIV prevalence developed by United Nations Joint Program on AIDS (UNAIDS). Since 2004, HSS data has been calibrated with Demographic and Health Survey and other indicators to determine national HIV prevalence[1].

Identifying sub-populations at high-risk for new HIV infection is a key to halting the spread of HIV within the population. Although current HIV diagnostic methods permit the calculation of HIV prevalence, this indicator provides a limited understanding of the most recent spread of infection. Accurate estimates of HIV incidence, which is the number of new infections over a defined period, in the population are needed. Such information will identify vulnerable populations and direct efficient targeted prevention programs and resources to the most at-risk subpopulations. The incidence data will also facilitate monitoring, appraise prevention efforts, detect sub-epidemics and track the occurrence of new waves of infection or disease[11]. Surveillance for HIV incidence provides a means to determine the proportion of new HIV-1 infections occurring in the population. Progress of the epidemic can then be tracked by these precise estimations of new burden of HIV infection.[11]

Newly developed assays offer opportunities to determine incidence of HIV in cross-sectional populations. These incidence assays are based on the underlying premise that the antibody production occurs months after HIV infection and that routine measurements of the different types of antibodies will help determine whether an infection has been recently acquired or not. These assays are however liable to misclassification of long-term infections as recent.

It is necessary to determine the population specific proportion of misclassified recent infections - the false recent rate (FRR) of these assays in order calculate HIV incidence- the proportion of persons infected with HIV, for a period less than 12 months.. The lower the FRR of an assay, the better it is for measuring HIV incidence in a population. This study was therefore carried out to estimate the false recent rate of two assays; the commercial BED HIV-1 (BED-CEIA) and the Limiting Antigen Avidity Assay among HIV patients in Ghana in order to determine a suitable assay for use in Ghana.

## Approach

This was a cross-sectional survey that involved long-term HIV infections in Ghana. Serum specimens were collected from eight clinical sites offering antiretroviral therapy (ART) services for HIV/AIDS from February 2010 to December 2010. The target group was consented patients aged 18 years or older with known HIV-positive status of at least 12 months without ART experience. A total of 1,045 specimens were collected from the eight sites. Any patients on ART, with HIV type-2, HIV-1/2 or indeterminate antibody results were excluded from the study. Hospital folder review was conducted to obtain data on age, risk factors for HIV infection, CD4 counts and opportunistic infections of the patients enrolled in the study. Two assays were then evaluated for their suitability to estimate HIV incidence in Ghana:

- The commercial BED HIV-1 incidence assay, which measures the levels of anti-HIV-1 IgG antibody relative to total IgG to distinguish persons with recent and long-term HIV infection.
- The limiting antigen avidity assay (LAg) developed by the United States Centers for Disease Surveillance and Prevention (CDC), Atlanta, measures the avidity of HIV-1 antibody to identify recent and long-term HIV infection.

The serum specimens were first tested by the BED assay at NMIMR, Legon and then shipped to the CDC Atlanta, for further BED and LAg testing. The false recent rate (FRR) of the BED and the LAg assays were then determined.

This study was a research collaboration between NMIMR, the National HIV AIDS Control Programme (NACP) of the Ghana Health Service and the Global AIDS Program Division of the United States Centres for Disease Control and Prevention (CDC). The study protocol was reviewed and approved by the Institutional review boards of the NMIMR, Legon and CDC, Atlanta.

## Results and Discussion

The results showed that the most dominant age group among the enrolled participants was 35-44 years (36%) whilst the common risk factor for HIV was a heterosexual partner (41%). The most prevalent opportunistic infection observed was candida (39%) and about 70% of the enrolled participants had CD4 cell counts less than 200 cells/mm$_3$. The BED FRR was estimated as 6.40% and the LAg FRR estimated as 0.74%. From this study, the BED assay was found to misclassify 6.4% of the study population as recent HIV infections compared to the LAg, which misclassified only 0.74% as recent HIV infections. Currently, there are no global reference standards. The general view is that the ability of an assay to classify individuals with long-standing infection as recently infected at a very low rate (low FRR) represents subsequent good utilisation for population studies to determine HIV incidence. From the results, the LAg has a lower misclassification rate of recent HIV infections in Ghana and is therefore a more suitable assay to measure HIV incidence. Due to the generalized nature of the HIV epidemic in Ghana, it has been proposed that the estimation of HIV incidence should focus on sub-populations of strategic importance and enable comparison of HIV incidence estimates in the same population for over a period of time. Target sub-populations for HIV incidence estimation will therefore include the most at risk groups such as female sex workers and men who have sex with men. Samples collected from pregnant women within the annual HSS could also be useful for HIV incidence estimations.

## Conclusion

The LAg assay could be used to estimate the HIV incidence rate in Ghana considering its low false recent rate. However, there is a need to define an appropriate study population for such an HIV incidence study and then use this population for subsequent years. This study has provided a valuable tool to guide considerations for assay-based HIV incidence surveillance in Ghana.

# 2. Serological profiling of HIV infected patients in Ghana

The accurate assessment of individuals infected with HIV and the differentiation of the type of infection, is essential in the evaluation of the current preventive efforts to restrict the spread of the virus to populations at risk.[11] The HIV and AIDS epidemic in Ghana has always been characterized by the co-circulation of HIV-1 and HIV-2.[12, 13,14] The majority of the infections being due to HIV-1,[3, 8] with HIV-2 and HIV-1/HIV-2 dual infections under 5%.[3,8,12,16] The trends of HIV-1 prevalence, estimated from the national HIV Sentinel Survey (HSS) in recent times have been 94.5% in 2008, 91.8% in 2009 and 96% in 2010.[3] Thus, although HIV-1 had been the predominant type, the proportion due to HIV-2 alone or HIV-1/2 dual infections had been unstable. Antiretroviral therapy (ART) was introduced in Ghana in 2003 and the programme has been rapidly scaled up with an estimated 42,000 patients on ART in 150 care centres in all ten regions of the country at the end of 2010.[17] This national programme uses standard first- and second-line regimens based on combinations of drugs from three drug classes: nucleoside reverse transcriptase inhibitors (NRTIs), non-nucleoside reverse transcriptase inhibitors (NNRTIs) and protease inhibitors (PIs).[18] Although HIV-2 is known to be naturally resistant to the NNRTI class of drugs,[19] patients on ART are usually put on the standard first-line regimen, which consists of NNRTI without first determining the type of HIV they are infected with.

In monitoring the emergence of HIV resistance to first-line antiretroviral use in Ghana, a drug resistance survey targeted at HIV-1 was set up by the National AIDS/Sexually Transmitted Infections (STI) Control Programme (NACP).[17] As these survey protocols target HIV-1 (the predominant type worldwide), it is important to determine the serotype of HIV infection prior to genotyping analyses. We therefore sought to determine the serological profile of these patients.

## Approach

Ten ART sites were selected based on the following criteria:

- Provision of ART had been available for at least three years within the survey area;
- Routine data collection as per national ART client record booklets;
- Laboratory capacity to initially process blood specimens.

The sites were Korle Bu Teaching Hospital, Accra; Komfo Anokye Teaching Hospital, Kumasi; Eastern Regional Hospital, Koforidua; Atua Government Hospital, Atua; St. Martins de Pores Hospital, Agomanya; Central Regional Hospital, Cape Coast; Effia Nkwanta Hospital, Sekondi; Brong Ahafo Regional Hospital, Sunyani; Holy Family Hospital, Techiman and Tamale Teaching Hospital, Tamale.

Whole blood samples were collected from patients at the start of first-line ART from the 10 sites between January 2008 and December 2010. These were processed to obtain plasma and tested onsite at the hospitals with rapid assays in accordance with the national guidelines on HIV. The blood samples were then transported in cold boxes with ice packs to the NMIMR within 48 hours. A line immunoblot assay, Inno-lia HIV-I/II Score (Innogentics, Belgium) was then applied to determine the presence of specific antibodies against HIV-1 and HIV-2. The INNO-LIA™ HIV I/II Score differentiates between HIV-1 and HIV-2 infections. The assay was performed following the manufacturer's instructions and the results were interpreted accordingly.[20]

## Results and Discussion

Out of the 1227 samples tested by the Inno-lia assay, 1174 (95.7%) were HIV-1, 13 (1%) were HIV-2 and 40 (3.3%) were HIV-1 and HIV-2 dual infections (Table 1). The prevalence of HIV-1 infection in the study population ranged from 89.1% in the Eastern Region to 100% each in the Brong Ahafo and Northern Regions. Out of the 13 HIV-2 infections found, seven (54%) were from the three sites located in the Eastern region (Atua Government, St. Martin de Porres and Eastern regional hospitals). (Table17. 1).

Table 17.1:   Distribution of HIV types among the study population for the various study sites

| Study site and Location | Number (%) of HIV types | | | Total |
|---|---|---|---|---|
| | HIV-1 | HIV-2 | HIV-1/2 | Number |
| Atua Government Hospital, Atua | 121 (93.1) | 1 (0.8) | 8 (6.2) | 130 |
| St. Martin de Pores Hospital, Agomanya | 114 (89.1) | 1 (0.8) | 13 (10.1) | 128 |
| Eastern Regional Hospital, Koforidua | 134 (93.7) | 5 (3.5) | 4 (2.8) | 143 |
| Korle Bu Teaching Hospital, Accra | 112 (96.6) | 0 (0) | 4 (3.4) | 116 |
| Central Regional Hospital, Cape-Coast | 129 (98.5) | 0 | 2 (1.5) | 131 |
| Efia-Nkwanta Hospital, Sekondi | 126 (97.0) | 2 (1.5) | 2 (1.5) | 130 |
| Brong Ahafo Regional Hospital, Sunyani | 113 (100) | 0 (0) | 0 (0) | 113 |
| Komfo Anokye Teaching Hospital, Kumasi | 119 (94.4) | 1 (0.8) | 6 (4.8) | 126 |
| Holy Family Hospital, Techiman | 106 (96.4) | 3 (2.7) | 1 (0.9) | 110 |
| Tamale Teaching Hospital, Tamale | 100 (100) | 0 (0) | 0(0) | 100 |
| Total | 1174 (95.7) | 13 (1) | 40 (3.3) | 1227 |

*HIV-1/2 infections represent samples that had antibodies to HIV-1 as well as antibodies to HIV-2*

The results obtained in this study were similar to those obtained from the 2010 HIV Sentinel Survey (HSS) conducted by the NACP. This study found 95.7% HIV-1 infections which is similar to the 96% HIV-1 infections obtained in the 2010 HSS.[21] However the proportions of samples that were HIV-2 only and those with HIV-1/2 dual infections were slightly different (1.4% for HIV-2 and 2.6% HIV-1/2 for the HSS compared to 1% HIV-2 and 3.3% HIV-1/2 in our study).

Our data also confirm the current predominance of HIV-1 infections in Ghana. However, there is a need to focus attention on those infected with HIV-2. Previous reports on HIV-1/2 dual infections showed that while ART reduced HIV-1 viral load, the viral load of the HIV-2 component continued to increase during therapy.[22] It is therefore likely that patients may experience early virologic failure if their regimen contains NNRTIs or the protease inhibitors. Three sites located in the Eastern region contributed more than half (54%) of the HIV-2 infections observed. About 64% of dual HIV infections were also found in the Eastern region. Thus, the Eastern region seems to bear the heaviest burden of HIV-2 infections. The Holy Family and Efia Nkwanta hospitals in the Brong Ahafo and Western regions respectively also had HIV-2 infections present either occurring singly or in combination with HIV-1 (Table 17.1). Although HIV-2 infections were not found in two of the study sites (Tamale Teaching and Brong Ahafo Regional hospitals), HIV-2 infections may be present throughout the country and are not confined to any region. This is because another site in the Brong Ahafo region (Holy Family hospital, Techiman) had 2.7% HIV-2 only and 0.9% being HIV-1/2 dual.

The standard first-line regimen for ART in Ghana consists of two drugs from the nucleoside reverse transcriptase inhibitor class and one drug from the NNRTI class. Patients infected with HIV-2 usually respond poorly to drugs from the NNRTI class and some protease inhibitors. [22, 23] It is therefore important to design special drug regimens for for such patients with HIV-2 infections. The use of HIV-2 viral load assays will also help greatly to monitor treatment outcomes in those infected with HIV-2 only or dual HIV-1 and HIV-2 infections.[22, 24]

## Conclusion

The results from this study confirm the co-existence of the two HIV types as indicated by the national HSS. Although HIV-1 infections are dominant (95.7%) in Ghana, our data shows the presence of HIV-2 occurring alone in 1% and in combination with HIV-1 in 3.3%. Therefore, it is important to determine the serotype of HIV infected patients before ART initiation. This will guide the choice of appropriate drugs in the first-line regimen for the HIV-2 infected patients. This will then optimize the benefits derived from ART by all patients and encourage proper monitoring for successful treatment outcomes and reduction of further transmission.

These two studies have contributed to the national response in the prevention and management of HIV infections in Ghana by (1) identifying an assay that can be used to measure HIV incidence and help track the epidemic and (2) estimating proportions of people infected with HIV-2 to inform special antiretroviral therapy regimen and monitoring.

## Acknowledgements

The authors would like to acknowledge all the study participants, the Ghana Health Service, the National AIDS/STI Control Program, the World Health Organization and the US Centers of Disease Control and Prevention for the support provided for the work described. The authors also acknowledge the immense contributions of Christopher Zaab-Yen Abana, Gifty Mawuli and all members of the HIV team in the Virology Department of NMIMR.

# References

1. National AIDS/STI Control Programme, Ghana Health Service, National HIV Prevalence and AIDS estimates report 2012-2016
2. Neequaye, A. R., Mingle, J. A., Neequaye, J. E. *et al.* A report of human immunodeficiency virus (HIV) infection in Ghana up to December 1986. *Ghana. Med. J.* 1987; 21:7-11.
3. National AIDS/STI Control Programme, Ghana Health Service, 2012 *HIV Sentinel Survey Report*, May 2013
4. Brandful, J., Ampofo, W., Apeagyei, F., Asare-Bediako, K., Osei-Kwasi, M., Predominance of human immunodeficiency virus type 1 among AIDS and AIDS-related complex patients in Ghana, West Africa, *East Afr Med. J.* 1997; 74: 17-20.
5. Kinomoto, M., Appiah-Opong, R., Brandful, J.A. *et al.* (2005). HIV-1 proteases from drug-naive West African patients are differentially less susceptible to protease inhibitors. Clin Infect Dis. 2005; 41: 243–251.
6. Delgado, E., Ampofo, W. K., Sierra, M. et al, High prevalence of unique recombinant forms of HIV-1 in Ghana: molecular epidemiology from an antiretroviral resistance study. *J. Acquir. Immun. Defic. Syndr.* 2008; 48:599-606.
7. Sagoe, K. W. C., Dwidar. M., Lartey, M. *et al.* Variability of the human immunodeficiency virus type 1 polymerase gene from treatment naïve patients in Accra, Ghana. *J Clin Virol.* 2007; 40:163–167
8. Brandful, J. A. M., Candotti, D. and Allain, J-P. Genotypic diversity and mutation profile of HIV-1 strains in antiretroviral treatment (ART) – Naïve Ghanaian patients and implications for antiretroviral treatment (ART). *J AIDS and HIV Res* 2012; 4(7): 187-197
9. Santos, A. F. and Soares, M. A. (2010). HIV Genetic Diversity and Drug Resistance, *Viruses* 2: 503-531.

10. Mastro, T. D., Kim, A. A., Hallett, T. *et al*, Estimating HIV Incidence in Populations Using Tests for Recent Infection: Issues, Challenges and the Way Forward. *J HIV AIDS Surveill Epidemiol.* 2010; 2(1):1-14. Epub 2010/01/01.

11. Mastro, T. D. Determining HIV Incidence in Populations: Moving in the Right Direction. *Journal of Infectious Diseases.* November 2012.

12. Bonney, E. Y., Sackey, S. T., Brandful, J. A. M., Laboratory diagnosis of dual HIV-1/HIV-2 infection in Ghanaian patients. *East Afr Med. J.* 2008; 85 (12): 534-543

13. Kawamura, M., Ishikawa, K., Mingle, J. A. A. *et al*, Immunological reactivities of Ghanaian sera with HIV-1, HIV-2 and simian immunodeficiency virus SIVagm, AIDS 1989; 3:609-611.

14. Hishida, O., Ayisi, N., Aidoo, M. *et al*. Serological survey of HIV-1, HIV-2 and human T-cell leukaemia virus type 1 for suspected AIDS cases in Ghana. AIDS. 1994; 8: 1257-1261

15. Takehisa, J., Osei-Kwasi, M., Ayisi, N. K. *et al* Phylogenetic analysis of HIV Type 2 in Ghana and Intrasubtype Recombination of HIV Type 2. *AIDS Res Hum Retrovir.* 1997; 13(7): 621-623

16. Ampofo, W., Koyanagi, Y., Brandful, J., Ishikawa, K., Yamamoto, N. Seroreactivity clarification and viral load quantification in HIV-1 and HIV-2 infections in Ghana. *J Med Dent Sci* 1999; 46 (1): 53-62.

17. National AIDS /STI Control Programme, Ghana Health Service, Protocol: HIV Drug Resistance Threshold Survey, 2006.

18. National AIDS/STI Control Programme; Ministry of Health; Ghana Health Service. Guidelines for antiretroviral therapy in Ghana, Ministry of Health 2010

19. Damond, F., Brun-Vezinet, F., Matheron, S. *et al,* Polymorphism of the Human Immunodeficiency Virus Type 2 (HIV-2) Protease Gene and Selection of Drug Resistance Mutations in HIV-2 patients treated with protease inhibitors. *J Clin Microbiol* 2006, 484-487.

20. User Manual, INNO-LIA$_{TM}$ HIV-I/II Score, Innogenetics, Belgium

21. National AIDS/STI Control Programme, Ghana Health Service. 2010 HIV Sentinel Survey Report, 2011.

22. Schutten, M., van der Ende, M. E, Osterhaus, A. D. M. E. Antiretroviral therapy in patients with dual infection with Human Immunodeficiency Virus types 1 and 2. *N Engl J M* 2000; 342 (2): 1758-1760

23. Adje-Toure, C., Cheingsong, R., Garcia-Lerma, J. *et al*. Antiretroviral therapy in HIV-2–infected patients: changes in plasma viral load, CD4+ cell counts, and drug resistance profiles of patients treated in Abidjan, Cote d'Ivoire. *AIDS* 2003; 17 (3):49–54.

24. Rode´s B., Carlos Toro, C., Jimenez, V. and Soriano, V. Viral response to antiretroviral therapy in a patient coinfected with HIV type 1 and 2. *CID* 2005; 41:e19-21

# Chapter 18
# The Role of the Polio Laboratory in Surveillance for Polio Eradication in Ghana

*John Kofi Odoom Jacob Barnor, Lindsay Forrest, Glynis Dunn, Miriam Eshun, William Kwabena Ampofo, Evangeline Obodai, Jacob Arthur-Quarm, Philip D. Minor and Javier Martin*

## Introduction

Poliovirus is the causative agent of paralytic poliomyelitis, a disease targeted by the World Health Organization (WHO) for eradication after the 1988 resolution by the World Health Assembly.[1, 2] Poliovirus is a human enterovirus (HEV) of species C belonging to the family *Picornaviridae*, a group of non-enveloped positive strand RNA viruses, and exists as three different serotypes, namely 1, 2 and 3, respectively. The coding region of the poliovirus genome is translated as a single polyprotein which is processed to generate the viral capsid (VP1 to VP4 proteins) and the nonstructural proteins. The genes coding for structural and nonstructural proteins are located at the 5' and 3' halves of the poliovirus genome, respectively. The coding region is preceded by a 5' noncoding region (NCR) of approximately 740 nucleotides organized in structural stem-loop domains important for RNA synthesis and translation initiation. The 3' end of the genome consists of an NCR of about 70 nucleotides which is also involved in RNA replication.[3] During their replication in humans, polioviruses accumulate mutations very rapidly due to the high error rate of the viral RNA-dependent RNA polymerase. Mutations accumulate sequentially during human infection at a nearly uniform rate of 1% to 2% nucleotide changes per year, acting as a molecular clock and making it possible to establish epidemiological and temporal links between polio cases.[4-6] In addition to a high mutation rate, genomic recombination is a common event during poliovirus evolution.[7,8]

The Global Polio Eradication Initiative (GPEI) followed a World Health Assembly resolution in 1988 with an aim to eradicate paralytic poliomyelitis by the year 2000.[9] The main strategies for the eradication programme are the use of extensive immunisation campaigns with live-attenuated oral polio vaccine (OPV) and the surveillance of acute flaccid paralysis (AFP) with clinical laboratory support. Although the year 2000 target was not met, considerable progress has been made towards interrupting the transmission of wild-type poliovirus globally, resulting in a reduction of more than 99% in the incidence of poliomyelitis worldwide and a decrease in the number of polio-endemic countries from 125 in 1988 to 4 in 2010.[10]

The search for poliomyelitis cases started in Ghana as early as 1976 when Ofosu-Amaah and colleagues did a survey in schools throughout the country. They estimated the prevalence of lameness attributed to poliomyelitis to be 5-8 per 100,000 school-aged children and an estimated mean annual incidence of paralytic poliomyelitis of 23 per 100,000 population.[11] The Expanded Programme on Immunisation (EPI) was introduced in Ghana in 1978, and has been operational in all regions of the country since 1985.[12] The GPEI programme was formally introduced in 1996 to intensify routine polio immunisation, implement supplementary immunisation activities (SIAs) such as national, sub-national, synchronized and mop-up immunisation campaigns. The national polio eradication initiative also established an active AFP surveillance for poliovirus with full laboratory support.[13] A number of performance indicators have been used to monitor the quality of AFP surveillance and the laboratory analysis is reviewed annually to assess the efficiency of isolation and characterization of poliovirus from AFP stool samples.[14]

The country has a medical officer in each district who is actively involved in the detection of all AFP cases. Weekly surveillance data are sent from all health centres to the National EPI office in Accra. The data are collected from any case of AFP in a child aged < 15 years without any other obvious cause or for any case of paralytic illness, regardless of patient's age, in which poliomyelitis is suspected. The data include details of the patient such as age, sex, location, immunization history and clinical symptoms. Other details including date of onset of paralysis, date of stool collection and date sent to the laboratory were also recorded.

This paper describes the molecular analysis of wild-type 1 poliovirus strains isolated in Ghana between 1995 and 2008, and non-polio enteroviruses (NPEVs) circulating among AFP patients and healthy school children. This is the first comprehensive study that covers the period between the establishment of AFP surveillance and supplementary immunization activities.

## Approach

### Virus isolation and typing

Faecal specimens from suspected AFP cases were processed at the National Polio Laboratory in Ghana according to WHO standard protocols. Thirteen L20B, HEp-2c and RD cell lines were used for virus isolation. Working poliovirus preparations were obtained by growth of the viruses in HEp-2C cells at 36°C in MEM without foetal calf serum. Isolates were typed by a neutralization assay, using standard antiserum pools supplied by the National Institute of Public Health and the Environment (RIVM), Bilthoven, The Netherlands. Intratypic differentiation (ITD) was done by two WHO-recommended methods: enzyme-linked immunosorbent assay (ELISA) using highly specific crossed-absorbed antisera and nucleic acid hybridization, a molecular method involving the use of genotype-specific nucleic acid probes.[13]

### Reverse transcription PCR and nucleotide sequencing of poliovirus genomes

Poliovirus RNA was purified from cell culture supernatants and used for reverse transcription polymerase chain reaction (RT-PCR) using standard procedures. The One-step RT-PCR kit (QIAGEN) was used to amplify three regions of the genome: 5'NCR (nt 68-530), the entire capsid protein VP1 coding region (nt 2479-3479), and a fragment of the non-structural coding region (nt 5844-6473) which included part of 3C and 3D genes. The purified viral RT-PCR DNA products were directly sequenced using the Big-Dye Terminator Cycle Sequencing (Applied Biosystems, Singapore) on the ABI Prism DNA 377 Sequencer as instructed by the manufacturer. Sequence data were stored as Standard Chromatogram Format (*.scf) files, analysed and edited using the Wisconsin Package Version 10.0-UNIX (GCG) and AlignIR V11 (LI-COR) software. The nucleotide sequence data reported in here are available from the EMBL Data Library under accession nos. JN393014 to JN393205.

## Sequence analysis

Phylogenetic relationships between strains were established by comparing their sequences after aligning them using the alignment program CLUSTAL X.[15] Phylogenetic relationships between sequences were inferred by the maximum likelihood method with DNADIST/ NEIGHBOR of PHYLIP (Phylogeny Inference Package) version 3.6 and a distance matrix was calculated using the F84 model of nucleotide substitution with a transition/transversion ratio (Ts/Tv) of 10.0. [16] The robustness of phylogenies was estimated by bootstrap analyses with 1,000 pseudoreplicate data sets generated with the SEQBOOT program of PHYLIP. Phylogenetic trees were constructed using neighbour-joining of PHYLIP and drawn using TREEVIEW or NJ Plot software.[17] The MEGA 3.1 software package was used to perform most of these analyses.

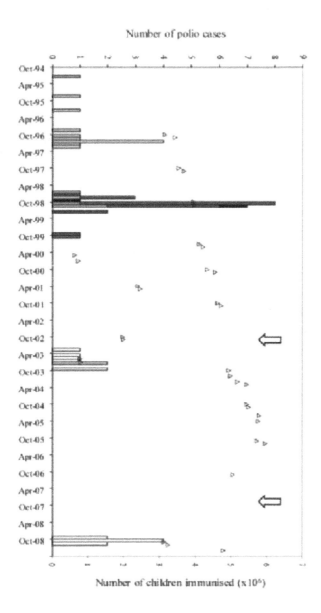

*Figure 18.1: Timeline of wild-type 1 poliovirus isolations in Ghana between 1995-2008. The number of polio cases is indicated by light grey (genotype I), dark grey (genotype II) and white (genotype III) bars. Triangles indicate the number of children immunised in NIDs or sub-NIDs. Arrows indicate gaps in immunisation.*

# Results and Discussion

## Polio immunization and cases

The number of children immunized with OPV from 1996 when supplemental immunization activities started in Ghana and the number of poliovirus cases isolated in the country are shown in Figure 18.1. The polio cases appeared to follow a seasonal distribution with peak between October and December just after the rainning season. However, all cases from 2003 occurred before the expected seasonal peak and did not follow the normal pattern.

The evolution of the AFP performance indicators in Ghana during the period of study showed low levels of performance during initial stages of the programme. The four northern regions, Brong Ahafo, Northern, Upper West, and Upper East, accounted for 28% of the total population of children under 15 years in Ghana but recorded only 13% and 5.2% of the total AFP cases in 1996 and 1997, respectively. From 1998 onwards, however, the numbers of AFP cases were more evenly distributed geographically. Consequently, most of the wild-type polioviruses isolated in Ghana during 1995–1997 (92.3%) came from southern districts (Figure 18. 2).

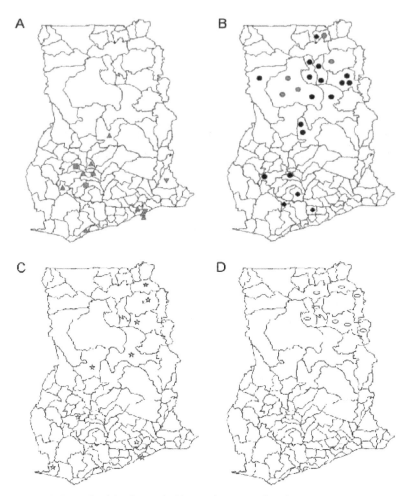

Figure 18.2: Geographical distribution of wild-type polio cases in Ghana between 1995-2008: A, 1995-1997; B, 1998-1999; C, 2003; D, 2008. Shapes indicate year of isolation, inverted triangle (1995), triangle (1996), square (1997), circle (1998), rhomboid (1999), star (2003) and ellipse (2008). Colours indicate genotype: light grey (I), dark grey (II) and white (III).

## Isolation of Poliovirus

The National Polio Laboratory processed approximately 4000 stool specimens between 1996 and 2008 that were collected from AFP cases through the active surveillance system in Ghana. From these samples, 56 wild-type 1, 99 Sabin-like polioviruses and 234 non-polio enteroviruses were isolated. Furthermore, from 1997 to 2003, approximately 2500 samples were collected from 2500 healthy children, and 15 wild-type 1, 65 Sabin-like polioviruses as well as 314 non-polio enteroviruses were isolated. Details of all AFP samples received in the polio laboratory with virus isolation from 1995-2011 and wild-type poliovirus isolations from 1995 to 2008 in Ghana are shown in Table 18.1.

Table 18.1.   Poliovirus and NPEV isolation from AFP samples in Ghana. (1995-2011)

| Year | No. of AFP cases | Wild  PV | Sabin-like | NPEV (%) |
|------|------------------|----------|------------|----------|
| 1995 | 5 | 2 | 0 | 0 |
| 1996 | 23 | 9 | 0 | 2 (8.7) |
| 1997 | 77 | 2 | 0 | 4 (5.2) |
| 1998 | 170 | 23 | 4 | 7 (4.1) |
| 1999 | 78 | 3 | 4 | 3 (3.8) |
| 2000 | 316 | 0 | 18 | 42 (13.3) |
| 2001 | 278 | 0 | 13 | 39 (14) |
| 2002 | 136 | 0 | 7 | 23 (16.9) |
| 2003 | 199 | 8 | 20 | 25 (12.6) |
| 2004 | 163 | 0 | 9 | 19 (11.7) |
| 2005 | 173 | 0 | 10 | 25 (14.5) |
| 2006 | 174 | 0 | 1 | 17 (9.8) |
| 2007 | 165 | 0 | 5 | 13 (8) |
| 2008 | 240 | 8 | 8 | 15 (6.3) |
| 2009 | 308 | 0 | 28 | 29 (9.4) |
| 2010 | 217 | 0 | 11 | 35 (16) |
| 2011 | 275 | 0 | 40 | 61 (22.2) |

## Phylogenetic Analysis of Wild-Type 1 Polioviruses from Ghana

A total of 63 wild-type 1 polioviruses were characterized. They represent 88.7% (63 of 71) of the total number of wild-type 1 viruses isolated in Ghana during the period of study. No wild-type 2 or 3 polioviruses were isolated in Ghana during 1995–2008. Comparisons of nucleotide sequence within the capsid VP1 coding region identified three different genotypes among the Ghanaian isolates. The viruses were related to African genotypes WEAF-A, -B and -C, which are the 3 genotypes that have circulated in Central and West Africa since the early 1990s.[19, 20] The three genotypes were named I, II, and III for the purpose of this study.

The two viruses from 1995 were relatively close to each other (2.59% sequence difference in VP1) but were distant from isolates of genotype I from subsequent years (between 8.58%-10.52% VP1 nucleotide differences). The other genotype I isolates grouped closely together (average VP1 sequence difference of 3.46%) (Fig.18.3B). The genotype I poliovirus isolates from 1996 showed an average VP1 sequence difference of 3.19%, while the average difference between genotype I isolates from 1998 was only 1.12%. Genotype II included viruses from 1998 and 1999, which were all very closely related and showed an average 1.40% nucleotide difference among them in the VP1sequence. All isolates from healthy and AFP cases from 2003 were phylogenetically close to each other (the average VP1 sequence difference between them was 1.32%) and belonged to a third genotype, genotype III, with very different VP1 sequences from viruses of genotypes I and II (17. 92% and 20.44% VP1 nucleotide differences, respectively). Isolates from 2008 belonged to genotype III and had an average VP1 sequence difference of 8.39% from 2003 isolates. Their VP1 nucleotide sequences were 18.15% and 20.01% different from viruses of genotypes I and II, respectively. Two poliovirus strains with six nucleotide differences between them in the VP1 coding region were isolated from case No. 64 in 2008. Representatives of the three genotypes identified above were selected and their VP1 sequences compared to those of other wild-type 1 poliovirus available in public databases.

Genotypes I and II isolates were classified within the WEAF-A and WEAF-C genotypes, respectively, which circulated in the African region in the late 1990s and early 2000s (Fig.18.3). They were first detected in southern Ghana during 1995-1997 and were not found in northern districts until 1998. However, it is likely that genotype WEAF-A polioviruses were also present in northern areas before 1998 but were not detected due to poor surveillance. A rapid improvement in AFP surveillance and effective immunization campaigns helped to quickly eliminate genotype WEAF-A from the southern regions, and viruses of this genotype were not detected here from May 1997 onwards. Similarly, viruses from genotype WEAF-C detected in Ghana from July 1998 had much lesser impact in the southern regions.

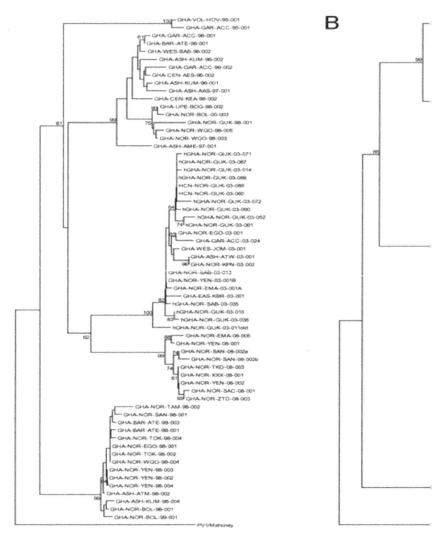

*Figure 18.3: Neighbour-joining trees representing phylogenetic relationships between the wild-type 1 poliovirus strains isolated in Ghana between 1995-2008. (A) 5'NCR (nucleotides 68-537). (B) VP1 coding region (nucleotides 2480-3385). (C) Partial 3CD coding region (nucleotides 5846-6478). Numbers at nodes indicate the percentage of 1,000 bootstrap pseudo replicates supporting the cluster. The sequences of PV1/Mahoney reference strain were introduced for correct rooting of the tree.*

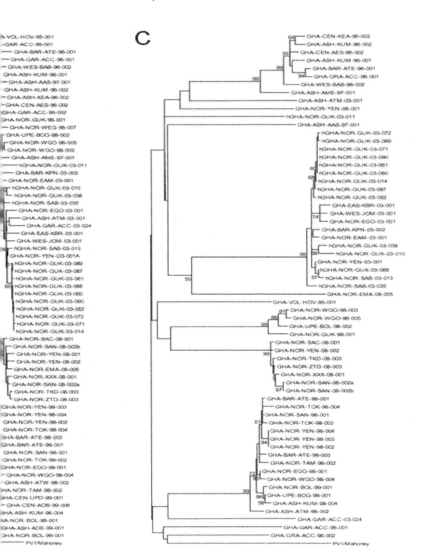

Both AFP surveillance and immunization rates reached high standards in the entire country soon after the 1998 epidemic, and only four viruses were detected in Ghana in 1999. However, wild-type 1 polioviruses were again found in Ghana in two separate outbreaks in 2003 and 2008 after long periods without polio cases. Viruses related to Ghanaian genotype III isolates seemed to have been well established in Central and West Africa well before the 2003 outbreak in Ghana, and the Ghanaian 2003 and 2008 strains were found to be closely related to several African isolates from 1999 to 2009. They all belong to the West Africa B (W EAF-B) genotype, which is still dominant in West and Central Africa. The Ghanaian isolates had no close genetic relationship with other wild-type 1 viruses identified in other parts of the world for which nucleotide sequences are publicly available.

It is likely that a decrease in population immunity against poliovirus due to reduced immnization campaigns played a significant role in the occurence of both the 2003 and 2008 outbreaks. Due to global programmatic priorities and a vaccine shortage, only one sub-National Immunization Day (NID) was carried out in Ghana in October 2002 and another in March 2003 when approximately 2 million and 0.8 million children, representing 44% and 17% of the target children respectively, were immunized. Similarly, only a single NID was conducted in Ghana in 2006 (November) that covered only 85% of the target group, while no NID was carried out in 2007. The most likely origin of both the 2003 and 2008 outbreaks in Ghana was Nigeria, where significant deficiencies in immunization and surveillance activities had been evident since 2002 and were responsible for large outbreaks that occurred between 2003 and 2008.[21-23]

### Recombination among wild-type 1 polioviruses from Ghana
Partial nucleotide sequences were also determined in 5' and 3'-end regions of the genome. The genetic relationships among isolates at the 5'NCR (Fig18.3a) were similar to those found when VP1 sequences were used. However, four major genetic groups were found in this instance with the two isolates from 1995 segregating as an independent cluster from their genotype I counterparts and showing large genetic

distances with respect to the rest of the viruses from genotype I and strains from genotype II and III.

As shown in Fig.18.3c, the phylogenetic tree constructed with 3CD sequences had a rather different topology. Five major genetic clusters can be clearly seen with viruses from genotype I splitting into two separate clusters, one including most isolates from 1996 and 1997 and the other comprising all isolates from 1998. Viruses from genotype III also split in two separate clusters, one including most isolates from 2003 and the other consisting of the majority of viruses from 2008. All strains from genotype II segregated as a separate group. Nine isolates, five from genotype I and four from genotype III (3 from 2003 and one from 2008), showed as separate single branches. They could not be assigned to any of the five genetic clusters. They contained 3CD sequences very different from each other and the rest of the Ghanaian isolates including those from contemporary viruses and/or strains of the same genotype. The sequence analysis indicated that frequent recombination events had likely occurred during the evolution of wild-type polioviruses in Ghana. The origin of the novel 3CD sequences is unclear. A blast search in Genebank using representatives of each of the 14 classes of 3CD sequences identified among the Ghanaian isolates showed that they were distantly related to type 1, 2 and 3 polioviruses including Sabin strains and wild-type poliovirus isolates and to members of species C HEVs prototype strains and isolates of different serotypes (Fig18.4A). However, as shown in Fig. 18.4B, despite the large number of nucleotide differences between them, all 14 classes of 3CD genomic sequences from Ghana clustered most closely with each other. They also showed some degree of genetic correlation with 3CD genomic sequences from two VDPV strains isolated in Nigeria in 2001 and 2002.

**A**

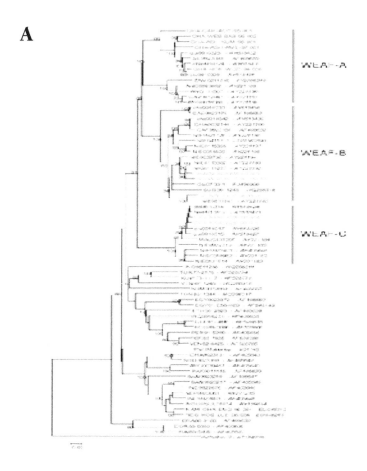

Figure 18.4: Neighbour-joining trees representing phylogenetic relationships between selected wild-type 1 poliovirus strains isolated in Ghana between 1995-2008 and other human enterovirus C strains isolated around the world. (A) VP1 coding region (nucleotides 2480-3385) of wild-type 1 polioviruses. (B) Partial 3CD coding region (nucleotides 5846-6478) of polio and non-polio human enterovirus C strains. Numbers at nodes indicate the percentage of 1,000 bootstrap pseudo replicates supporting the cluster. Selected wild-type 1 strains from Ghana are shown in red (genotype I), green (genotype II) and blue (genotype III). The position of isolates from West Africa genotypes A, B and C (WEAF-A, WEAF-B and WEAF-C, respectively) are shown in the tree.

**D**

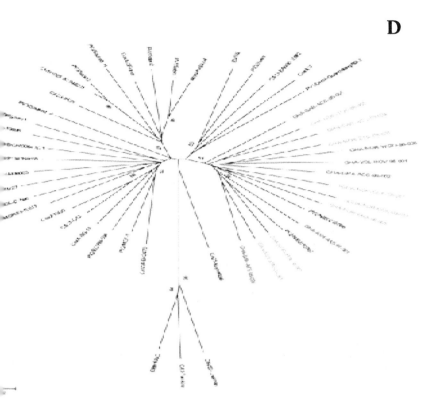

The possibility cannot be ruled out that the observed 3CD sequences were derived from other wild-type poliovirus strains. The occurrence of 14 different 3CD sequences among the wild-type isolates would mean that the number of circulating genotypes in Ghana were higher than the three observed from 1995-2008.

The results shown here clearly demonstrate that eradication of poliovirus is achievable if there is an efficient AFP surveillance system in place, as well as the implementation of high-quality, rapid, and efficient SIA immunization campaigns. Our results illustrate the impact of AFP surveillance during the early years of polio eradication efforts in Ghana, the importance of national immunization days (NIDs), and mop-up campaigns to eliminate wild-type poliovirus circulation and the risks of importation of wild-type poliovirus from other countries in the absence of high population immunity. Overall, the elimination of poliovirus circulation in Ghana can be considered a success, even in a context where neighboring countries have maintained or reestablished wild-type poliovirus endemicity, and would suggest that changing from a polio eradication effort to a control strategy[24] is not optimal, particularly in areas where maintaining high levels of routine immunization remains a challenge and GPEI strategies appear to be the best means to fight and eliminate this deadly disease.

## Non-polio enteroviruses

Non polio enteroviruses, NPEVs were found with an isolation rate between 8.4-11% among the AFP patients and 16.6 - 20% in the healthy children. The NPEV rate is a useful indicator of laboratory performance but may be influenced by a number of factors, including the season of the year, elevation, or population hygienic levels. Our studies identified Coxsackie B viruses to be most predominant NPEV in circulation among both AFP patients and healthy children. Apart from Cox B, E11and E6 were the next most prevalent strains in the AFP and healthy children respectively. Among the enteroviruses isolated in the healthy children, 15 turned out to be wild polioviruses from Gushegu in the Northern Region.

The majority of the NPEVs from both AFP cases and healthy children were untypable. The large number of unidentified NPEVs which could not be typed using the standard antisera contained in the kit is a limitation on the choice of assay. Therefore, molecular methods should be used in further classification of these viruses. Aggregated forms of NPEVs, reoviruses or adenoviruses could also not be ruled out.[25] According to reports, serum raised against one serotype does not cross-neutralize others, but serotypes can undergo some antigenic variation and limited neutralization is speculated to occur between several serotypes.[26]

In conclusion, wild polioviruses that circulated in Ghana between 1995 and 2008 belonged to the African genotypes WEAF-A, B and C. Our study also revealed that healthy children can harbour wild polioviruses without showing any paralysis. It is therefore essential that Ghana continues to maintain high vaccination coverage and a sensitive surveillance system to rapidly detect and respond to cases of suspected paralytic poliomyelitis, from indigenous sources, imported virus and from possible breaches in laboratory containment. Poliovirus from any of these sources entering the Ghanaian communities with low vaccine coverage may result in endemic or epidemic transmission.

## Acknowledgments

We thank Cara C. Burns for providing VP1 sequence data for some isolates and for helpful advice. We are also grateful to Mr. Kwame Domedah for his role in the laboratory. This study was supported by the Noguchi Memorial Institute for Medical Research and the National Institute for Biological Standards and Control (NIBSC) and the World Health Organisation (WHO).

## References

1. Dowdle, W. R., Featherstone, D. A., Birmingham, M. E., Hull, H. F. and Aylward, R. B. 1999. Poliomyelitis eradication. *Virus Res* 62:185-92.
2. Minor, P. D. 2004. Polio eradication, cessation of vaccination and re-emergence of disease. *Nat Rev Microbiol 2*: 473-82.
3. Minor, P. D. 1997. Poliovirus, p. 555-573. In: Nathanson N. ed. *Viral Pathogenesis,* Philadelphia: Lippincott-Raven Publishers.

4. Gavrilin, G. V., Cherkasova, E. A., Lipskaya, G. Y., Kew, O. M. and Agol, V.I. 2000. Evolution of circulating wild poliovirus and of vaccine-derived poliovirus in an immunodeficient patient: a unifying model. *J Virol* 74:7381-90.

5. Kew, O. M., Mulders, M. N., Lipskaya, G. Y., da Silva, E. E. and Pallansch, M. A. 1995. Molecular epidemiology of polioviruses. *Semin. Virol.* 6:401-414.

6. Martin, J. 2006. Vaccine-derived poliovirus from long term excretors and the end game of polio eradication. *Biologicals* 34: 117-22.

7. Cherkasova, E. A., Korotkova, E. A., Yakovenko, M. L., Ivanova,O. E., Eremeeva, T. P., Chumakov, K. M. and Agol, V. I. 2002. Long-term circulation of vaccine-derived poliovirus that causes paralytic disease. *J Virol* 76:6791-9.

8. Guillot, S., Caro, V., Cuervo, N., Korotkova, E., Combiescu, M., Persu, A., Aubert-Combiescu, A., Delpeyroux, F. and Crainic, R. 2000. Natural genetic exchanges between vaccine and wild poliovirus strains in humans. *J Virol* 74: 8434-43.

9. World Health Assembly. 1988. Eradication of poliomyelitis by the year 2000: resolution of the World Health Assembly. Geneva: World Health Organization (WHA resolution 41.28).

10. World Health Organization 2011, posting date. Global Polio Eradication Initiative. Monthly situation reports. [Online].

11. Ofosu-Amaah, S., J. H. Kratzer, and D. D. Nicholas. 1977. Is poliomyelitis a serious problem in developing countries?--lameness in Ghanaian schools. *Br Med J* 1: 1012-4.

12. Kim-Farley, R. 1992. Global immunization. The Expanded Programme on Immunization Team. *Annu Rev Public Health* 13: 223-37.

13. World Health Organization. 2004. Manual for the virological investigation of poliomyelitis. WHO/EP/GEN. W.H.O.

14. Centers for Disease Control and Prevention. Tracking progress toward global polio eradication--worldwide, 2009-2010. *MMWR Morb Mortal Wkly Rep* 60:441-5.

15. Thompson, J. D., Gibson, T. J., Plewniak, F., Jeanmougin, F. and Higgins, D. G.. 1997. The CLUSTAL_X windows interface: flexible strategies for multiple sequence alignment aided by quality analysis tools. *Nucleic Acids Res* 25:4876-82.

16. Felsenstein, J. 2000. PHYLIP: phylogeny inference package, version 3.6a3 (computer program). Distributed by the author, Department of Genetics. University of Washington, Seattle.

17. Perriere, G., and Gouy, M.1996. WWW-query: an on-line retrieval system for biological sequence banks. *Biochimie* 78:364-9.
18. World Health Organization. WHO vaccine-preventable diseases: monitoring system. 2011 global summary. Available at http://apps.who.int/immunization_monitoring/en/globalsummary/timeseries/tscoveragebcg.htm. Accessed 11 April 2012.
19. Gouandjika-Vasilache, I., Burns, C. C., Gumede, N., Guillot, S., Menard, D., Dosseh, A., Akoua-Koffi, C., Pallansch, M. A., Kew, O. M., and Delpeyroux, F. Delpeyroux. 2008. Molecular epidemiology of wild poliovirus type 1 circulation in West and Central Africa, from 1997 to 1999, using genotyping with a restriction fragment length polymorphism assay. *Arch Virol* 153: 409-16.
20. Morvan, J. M.,Chezzi, C., Gouandjika, I., Reimerink, J. H. and van der Avoort, H. G. 1997. The molecular epidemiology of type 1 poliovirus in Central African Republic. *J Gen Virol* 78 (Pt 3): 591-9.
21. World Health Organization. Progress towards the global eradication of poliomyelitis 2002. *Wkly Epidemiol Record* 2003; 78:138–44.
22. Centers for Disease Control and Prevention. Global Polio Eradication Initiative Strategic Plan, 2004. *MMWR Morb Mortal Wkly Rep* 2004; 53:107–8.
23. Olufowote, J. O. 2011. Local Resistance to the Global Eradication of Polio: Newspaper Coverage of the 2003-2004 Vaccination Stoppage in Northern Nigeria. *Health Commun.* 26(8):743-53
24. Arita, I., M. Nakane, and F. Fenner. 2006. Public health. Is polio eradication realistic? *Science,* 312:852-4.
25. Assad, F. and Cockburn, W. C. 1972 Four year study of WHO Virus reports on enteroviruses other than poliovirus. *Bull WHO.* 46: 329-339.
26. Introduction of Real Time RT-PCR into the Global Polio Laboratory Network. Available at: http://www.polioeradication.org/Research/PolioPipeline/No2Autumn2008/IntroductionofRealTimeRTPCR. Accessed on 20 Feb 2012.

# Chapter 19
## Investigations of Viral Haemorrhagic Fever Infections in Ghana

*Joseph H.K. Bonney, Mubarak Osei-Kwasi, Theophilus Adiku,*
*Jacob S. Barnor, Meike Pahmann, Robert Amesiya, Chrysanto*
*Kubio,Shirley Nimo Paintsil, Lawson Ahadzie, Stephan*
*Gunther and Wiiliam K Ampofo.*

## Introduction

Viral haemorrhagic fevers (VHFs) are a group of febrile highly infectious illnesses, and often fatal diseases caused by several viral families. They are characterized by the sudden onset of fever, malaise, headache, sore throat, abdominal pain, vomiting and bloody diarrhoea, skin rash, mucosal and gastrointestinal (GI) bleeding, oedema, and hypotension. The fatality rate varies depending on the infecting virus, but can be as high as 90 per cent.[1-3] There are four viral families known to cause VHF disease in humans; these are the *Arenaviridae, Bunyaviridae, Filoviridae, and Flaviviridae.* The viruses are usually transmitted by the bite of infected ticks and mosquitoes. Infection may also be transmitted between humans through contact with body fluids (e.g., blood, semen, urine) and possibly through droplets released into the air by coughing or sneezing.

Epidemics caused by haemorrhagic fever viruses, include Ebola, Marburg, Lassa fever,(LF) Crimean-Congo, Rift Valley fever, Yellow fever (YF), Dengue haemorrhagic fever (DHF) and Dengue (DEN) fever. Animal reservoirs including bats, rodents, ticks and mosquitoes pose a significant public health problem in the tropics.[4,5] In 1995, Le Guenno and colleagues, isolated and identified a new strain of Ebola virus from a single non-fatal human case in Côte d'Ivoire[6] and in the same year, an outbreak of Ebola haemorrhagic fever occurred in and around Kikwit, Democratic Republic of Congo with a fatality rate of 92%.[7] The isolation and identification of new viral strains in the family *Arenaviredae Lujo virus and Merino Walk virus* have recently been reported from South Africa.[8,9] Viral haemorrhagic fevers have been prominent among infectious diseases that have re-emerged in the last three decades.[10,12] The more recent outbreaks of Ebola haemorrhagic fever in the Isiro area in Democratic Republic of Congo and Kibaale district of Uganda,[13] with their associated high mortality rates, raised public health concerns, although VHFs have not been given the much needed attention. Lassa virus, for example, has been documented to occur in humans in most of West Africa and infects approximately 100,000 to 300,000 people every year, with an overall mortality rate ranging from 1% to 2%.[14,15] The World Health Organization (WHO) has classified LF as endemic in Nigeria, Sierra Leone and Liberia. In other West African countries including Côte d'Ivoire, Senegal, Guinea, Gambia, Burkina Faso, Mali and the Central African Republic, there has been documented incidence of LF and other haemorrhagic fever viruses such as Ebola.[15,16]

Most of the VHFs that are known to be endemic in the African region have not been documented in Ghana, although the reservoir hosts for most of them are widely distributed. For example, there is a paucity of information on Lassa fever in Ghana despite the widespread availability of the reservoir host, *Mastomys* rodents, in the country. In 2000 there was a report of a 23-year old German student tourist who died from LF after visiting Ghana, Côte d'Ivoire and Burkina Faso[17]. In the same year, four cases of new Lassa virus strains were imported into Germany and the United Kingdom by persons who had visited Ghana, Côte d'Ivoire, and Burkina Faso.[17,18] This raised questions regarding the probable circulation of LF and possibly other haemorrhagic fever viruses in Ghana. There have been speculations about the existence and occurrence of clinical cases of unrecognised haemorrhagic fever viruses over the years with particular reference to the Northern Region.

Yellow fever outbreaks are known to occur every 10 to 12 years in Ghana.[19] Three major outbreaks which affected different parts of the country occurred in 1969-70, 1977-80 and 1982-83 these together caused more than 400 deaths.[20] Sporadic epidemics of yellow fever virus infections have since been confirmed in areas where mostly irrigation is used for dry season farming as well as villages with large ponds serving as water reservoirs.[21] This notwithstanding, between 1997 and 2009, suspected yellow fever cases reported from various parts of Ghana were not confirmed by laboratory investigations with serological assays.[31,35] It was thus evident, that there could be haemorrhagic fevers in the country with the causative agents yet to be clearly identified.

The scarcity of data on haemorrhagic fevers in the country was in part due to the lack of laboratory diagnostic tools within Ghana Health Service facilities to fully profile suspected cases. Moreover, there have been few research projects seeking to identify and characterize aetiological agents of VHF, and estimate the disease burden. Suspected VHF cases submitted to national health laboratories are only tested serologically for yellow fever. These cases are not screened for VHF pathogens endemic in the African region and other viral infections such as viral hepatitis A, B, C and E that share similar symptoms. Thus most cases that presents with signs and symptoms suggestive of VHF/ yellow fever are not diagnosed, which leads to high mortality rates, probably due to poor case management.

There was therefore the need to establish differential diagnostic system to test for VHF pathogens endemic in Africa region and other viral infections with similar clinical presentations. Consequently, we initiated a study in 2010 which sought to detect and characterize agents of haemorrhagic fevers and viral hepatitis using serological and molecular tools, with particular interest in northern Ghana.

# Approach

## Study sites

Sixteen health facilities in the four regions of northern Ghana were chosen as study sites. These were in: Atebubu, Yeji, Techiman and Kwame Danso in the Brong-Ahafo Region; Damongo, Salaga, Yendi, Bole, Nalerigu, Gushiegu, Chereponi and Saboba in the Northern Region; Wa, Kaleo and Nandom in the Upper West Region and Bongo in the Upper East Region. The sites were selected on the basis of previous history of outbreaks and suspected of yellow fever. Some of the towns also share borders with countries where VHFs have been reported in the past. Most of these areas are characterized by a prolonged dry season and a short rainy season of five months, with annual rainfall under 900mm. Damongo in the West Gonja District in the Northern Region is approximately 30km from Mole, the biggest game reserve in the country. The game reserve covers about 300km² and harbours different species of animals including primates such as chimpanzees, baboons, African green monkeys and others with the potential of zoonotic spread of some VHFs.

## Study population

Study participants enrolled were VHF or viral hepatitis suspected patients without any gender or age bias who meet the case definition. The criteria used for enrolling patients included any person with severe illness, fever $\geq 38°C$, and at least one of the following signs: bloody stools, vomiting blood, unexplained bleeding from the mucosa, jaundice (yellow eyes, elevated serum bilirubin, or bilirubin in the urine), encephalitis (confusion, disorientation, drowsiness, convulsions), renal involvement (lower urine output, proteinuria, bloody urine), and abdominal pain with the absence of malaria and lack of response to antibiotics.

## Sample collection

Paired blood specimen was obtained from suspected cases – immediately when a case was suspected, and after 14 days or just before the patient was discharged. At each instance, 5 ml of whole blood was collected by venipuncture into a blood-collecting tube and labelled with patient identification and collection date. The patient's clinical and demographic details were also recorded on the case investigation form. Whole blood was then centrifuged at 1000 x g for 10 minutes to separate the serum which was then dispensed into two separate vials of approximately 1ml each and labelled appropriately. Where there was no centrifuge, blood was kept in the refrigerator at 4–8°C until there was complete retraction of the clot from the serum, then the serum carefully removed without extracting red cells. The serum was kept at 4–8°C either in a refrigerator or cool box with ice packs until shipment to the laboratory within seven days. Freezing of the specimens at this stage was avoided. In the laboratory, aliquots of sera were stored at -20°C.

Prior to sample collection, clinicians and other field staff were educated on the importance of adhering to strict biosafety guidelines for handling samples for their own safety and protection. Additionally, medical personnel trained in sample collection were urged to ensure that they follow standard precautions such as the use of barrier protection and other appropriate personal protective equipment during the manipulation of all specimens.

## Laboratory analysis

Clinical specimens were analysed by both serological and molecular assays. The serological techniques used include indirect immuno-fluorescence, enzyme-linked immunosorbent assay (ELISA) and particle agglutination assays. All the serological testing for the four unrelated hepatotropic viruses, Hepatitis A virus, (HAV), Hepatitis B virus (HBV), Hepatitis C virus (HCV) and Hepatitis E virus (HEV) which commonly causes viral hepatitis were done with ELISA. For hepatitis A, clinical serum samples were evaluated for the detection of anti-HAV antibodies. The kit used, HAV IgM ELISA (DRG, Ref: EIA-4432, Marburg, Germany), detects IgM class antibodies to HAV. Test screening for samples were carried out according to the manufacturer's instructions.

Two serological test assays were used in detection of hepatitis B surface antigen (HbsAg) and IgM class antibody to hepatitis B virus core antigen (HBc) in the clinical serum samples. Co-infection with hepatitis Delta was not evaluated. Laboratory investigations for HbsAg were done with HbsAgone, version ULTRA (DIA.PRO, Ref: SAGIULTRA.CE, Milano, Italy), and detection of IgM class antibody to HBc in the clinical sera was assayed with HBc IgM (DIA.PRO, Ref: BCM.CE, Milano, Italy). The screenings for the two tests were carried out according to the manufacturer's instructions.

Clinical serum samples were evaluated for the detection of anti-HCV IgM antibodies. The screening kit used, SERODIA®-HCV (Fujirebio Inc., Ref: BG05TE, Tokyo, Japan), was a particle-agglutination assay using gelatin particles coated with recombinant HCV antigens for the detection of antibodies to HCV in human serum and plasma. The assay used for the IgG test screening for HEV was an EIA kit with recombinant HEV antigens, recomWell HEV IgG (Mikrogen Diagnostik, Ref: 5004, Neuried, Germany), and the assay used for the IgM test screening was recomWell HEV IgM (Mikrogen Diagnostik, Ref: 5005, Neuried, Germany). A confirmatory test screening for the anti-HEV IgG and IgM antibodies was performed with recomLine (Mikrogen Diagnostik, Ref 5072, Neuried, Germany), an immunoblotting assay which uses recombinant purified antigens applied onto a nitrocellulose matrix membrane cut into strips.

Different techniques were used for different pathogens depending on the suitability and all protocols were followed according to the manufacturer's instructions. Various types of reverse transcription -polymerase chain reaction (RT-PCR) assays were performed for molecular detection of the different viral pathogens for viral hepatitis and VHFs in the clinical sera. The RT-PCR assays include conventional, modified conventional (nested and/or semi-nested) and real time reverse transcription (rRT). In addition a commercially manufactured PCR kit (Astra Diagnostics GmbH, Hamburg, Germany) for viral hepatitis was used to re-test all the clinical specimens investigated. Amplicons from positive specimens were purified on columns (Quick-SpinTM Qiagen, Hilden, Germany) and sequenced for further phylogenetic analysis.

# Results

In all, a total of 276 clinical specimens screened were analysed and each of the 16 study sites provided at least one clinical specimen. Of the total clinical specimens screened, 254 were analysed for gender and age. Males were in the majority (172; 68%) and of these, 84 (63.2%) tested positive for at least viral pathogens. Clinical specimens from females from all study sites numbered 82 of which 49 (59.8%) were positive for viral hepatitis and/or viral haemorrhagic fevers. The highest number of clinical specimens was obtained from children in the aged ≤10 years (41.3%) while the lowest number of specimens came from the 61 years and above (2.8%). Majority, 47 (44.8%) of the patients evaluated in the age category less than 10 years were found to be positive for the viral pathogens investigated whilst the elderly in the 60 years and above age group had the lowest number of positive cases-- 5 or (3.8%). A significant majority of 132 (52.0%) of all clinical specimens investigated for viral infections of hepatitis and haemorrhagic fevers were found positive for viral hepatitis and 12 (4.3%) for VHFs (p < 0.001).

The serological tests performed showed that 25 (9.1%) of all clinical specimens had detectable IgM antibodies against HAV. Surface antigen of hepatitis B virus (HbsAg) was detected in 103 (37.3%) whilst 29 (10.5%) of clinical specimens had immunoglobulin M (IgM) antibodies against HBV core antigen (anti-HBc Ag). Anti-HCV IgM antibodies were detected in 34 (12.3%) of screened clinical specimens. HEV enzyme immunosorbent assays initially detected anti-HEV immunoglobulin g (IgG) in 38 (13.8%) and IgM antibodies in 82 (29.7%). Further analysis with a line immunoblotting assay confirmed 30 (10.9%) and 64 (23.2%) of the specimens to be IgG and IgM positive respectively. Among the VHFs, detection of Dengue 2 IgM antibodies was the highest in all clinical specimens. Eight (2.9%) were positive for dengue 2 IgM whilst anti-Lassa and anti-Chikungunya IgG and IgM antibodies 2 (0.4%) was detected respectively.

Of all clinical specimens tested for viral hepatitis (276) by PCR, 31% were positive for HBV 23% HCV and 10% HAV. There were no positive signals with the various PCR used in the study for hepatitis E virus and all the VHFs investigated. Reverse transcription (RT)-PCR analysis and the Gel-based assay for HAV and HCV resulted in 21 and 23 positives respectively. Sixty four (23.2%), and 58 (21%) of the clinical specimens tested HBV positive by RT and conventional PCR respectively.

## Discussion

This study sought to investigate with serological and PCR-based assays the likely existence of haemorrhagic fever viruses in northern Ghana. Data generated from our study suggests that viral hepatitis, which shares clinical symptoms with VHFs, was widespread in the study area. Out of the total number of 172 male specimens analysed, 63% were positive for VHFs and viral hepatitis as against 37% for females. It has been established that males and females differ in their susceptibility to a diverse array of viral infections.[22] Vulnerability to viral infections is often lower among females because they typically mount stronger immune responses than males. Inborn identification and reaction to viruses differ between males and females during viral infections. This often results in gender differences in cytokine responses to infections that play a critical role in determining susceptibility to viruses.[22] Immune responses to viruses can differ with changes in hormone concentrations caused by natural fluctuations over the menstrual or oestrous cycle, from contraception use and during pregnancy.[23] While behavioural factors such as eating habits can influence exposure to viruses, several studies demonstrate that physiological differences between males and females cause dimorphic responses to infections.[22]

A relatively higher proportion of 35.3% (p = 0.20) from infants, pre- and school age groups (children less than 10 years) screened, tested positive for viral hepatitis and VHFs. As documented in various studies, age plays a critical role in determining viral virulence.[24,25] Many viral infections are far more severe in younger than in older hosts.[26] This increase in severity often correlates with increased replication and dissemination of the virus. The mechanism(s) are incompletely understood. It is commonly considered that maturation of the immune system explains increased resistance to viral infection in older hosts, but this has not been thoroughly confirmed. Other differences in cellular differentiation and proliferation may play a role. For instance, the genes expressed in the nervous system during infection of younger host's differ,[24] indicating that fundamental differences control how younger and older tissues respond to viral infection.

A significantly higher proportion of the samples were positive for viral hepatitis (52%) than VHFs (4%). These findings are consistent with previous studies done in Ghana where viral hepatitis and some haemorrhagic fever viruses were found to be endemic by the World Health Organisation (WHO).[21, 27] The sero-prevalence rate of chronic viral hepatitis among jaundiced patients in Ghana has been reported to be 54% [29] whilst a sero-positivity of 4% was found for Lassa fever.[29] There have been epidemics of agents of VHFs including yellow fever, especially in northern Ghana,[30-31] which support the recurrence and emergence of some agents of VHFs within specified time periods. A typical example is yellow fever which is endemic in Ghana but epidemics have been established to recur in every 10 to 12 years.[19] However, as recent as November 2011, three regions (Upper West, Northern and Greater Accra) were affected by yellow fever, with eight cases, three of which were laboratory confirmed. There were seven deaths reported by yellow fever surveillance teams. These deaths presented the clinical syndrome of fever and jaundice. Subsequent to this, the Ministry of Health declared a yellow fever outbreak in the country. The disease spread over to 8 of Ghana's 10 regions. By March 2012, preventive vaccination had helped to reduce the number of new cases and deaths.[32]

Viral hepatitis infections have been endemic in Ghana. There has been speculation, as yet unproven, that incidence rates of viral hepatitis increase from the southern to the northern parts of Ghana. However, regional figures from the Disease Surveillance Division of the GHS from 2004 to 2010 do not show are latively higher incidence of reported VH in the northern sector, but rather indicate its widespread occurrence all over the country.[33]

# Conclusion

Our findings indicate the possible circulation of Lassa, Dengue type 2 and Chikungunya viruses in Ghana. Our investigations do not indicate a significant presence of VHF agents in Ghana. However, the data suggest that viral hepatitis infections, which often share clinical symptoms with VHFs, are widespread, illustrating the need for differential diagnosis to be implemented. Further studies, which include animal vectors of VHFs such as Lassa fever, are underway to cover other regions of Ghana and provide more information on these dangerous zoonotic infections in the interest of public health.

# References

1.  Bannister, B. Viral haemorrhagic fevers imported into non-endemic countries: risk assessment and management. *B Med Bull..* 2010; 95(1): 193-225.

2.  Beeching, N. J., Fletcher, T. E. *et al.* Travellers and viral haemorrhagic fevers: what are the risks? *Int J Antimicro Agents.* 2010; 36: S26-S35.

3.  Fleischer, K.B., Kohler, *et al.* Lassa fever. *Med Klin* (Munich). 2000; 95(6): 340-345.

4.  Halstead, S. B. Dengue haemorrhagic fever - a public health problem and a field for research. *Bull WHO.* 1980; 58: 1-21.

5.  Monath, T.P. *Aedes albopictus*, an exotic mosquito vector in the United States. *Ann Intern Med.* 1986 Sep; 105 (3): 449-51.

6.  Le Guenno, B., Formenty, P. *et al.* Isolation and partial characterisation of a new strain of Ebola virus. *Lancet* 1995; (345): 1271-4

7.  Khan, A. S., Tshioko, F. K., Heymann, D. L. *et al.* The reemergence of Ebola haemorrhagic fever, Democratic Republic of the Congo, 1995. *J Infect Dis.* 1999; (179) S76-86.

8.  Briese, T. J., Paweska, T. *et al.* Genetic detection and characterization of Lujo virus, a new hemorrhagic fever-associated arenavirus from southern Africa. *PLoS Pathog.* 2009; 5(5): e1000455.

9.  Palacios, G., Savji, N. *et al.* Genomic and phylogenetic characterization of Merino Walk virus, a novel arenavirus isolated in South Africa. *J Gen Virol.* 2010; 91(5): 1315-1324.

10. Gubler, D. J. The global resurgence of arboviral diseases. *Trans Roy Soc Trop Med Hyg.* 1996; 90: 449-451

11. Bajani, M. D., Tomori, O., Rollin, P.E. *et al.* A survey for Lassa virus antibodies among health workers in Nigeria. *Trans Roy Soc Trop Med Hyg.* 1997; 91: 379-381.

12. Tukei, P. M. Threat of Marburg and Ebola viral haemorrhagic fevers in Africa. *East Afr Med J.* 1996; 73(1). P 27-31.

13. Centers for Disease Control and Prevention (CDC), Special Pathogens Unit. Available at: http://www.cdc.gov/ncidod/dvrd/spb/outbreaks/index.htm#ebola-drc-2012; Accessed on October 1, 2012.

14. Leparc-Goffart, I., Emonet, S.F. An update on Lassa virus. *Med Trop* (Mars). 2011; 71(6): 541-545.

15. Frame. J. D. Surveillance of Lassa fever in missionaries stationed in West Africa, *Bull WHO.* 1975; 52: 593-598.

16. Monath, T. P. Lassa fever: Review of epidemiology and epizootiology. *Bull WHO*. 1975; 52: 77-592.

17. Gunther, S., Emmerich, P. *et al*. Imported Lassa fever in Germany: molecular characterization of a new Lassa virus strain. *Emerg Infect Dis*. 2000; 6: 466-76.

18. Centers for Disease Control and Prevention/National Institutes of Health. *Biosafety in Microbiological and Biomedical Laboratories*. 4th Edition, Washington DC: U.S. Government Printing office. DHHS Publication CDC. 1999; 93 – 8395.

19. Addy, P. A. K., Minami, K. *et al*. Recent yellow fever epidemics in Ghana, 1969-1983. *East Afr Med J*. 1986; 63(6):422-433

20. Ghana – W.H.O. Available at: www.who.int/entity/csr/disease/yellowfev/ghana_en.pdf. Date accessed: October 1, 2012.

21. Appawu, M. and Dadzie, S. *et al*. Surveillance of viral haemorrhagic fevers in Ghana: entomological assessment of the risk of transmission in the northern Regions. *Ghana Med J*. 2006; 40(4):137-141.

22. Klein, S. L., Jedlicka, A., Pekosz, A. The Xs and Ys of immune responses to viral vaccines. *Lancet Infect Dis*. 2010; 10(5): 338-49.

23. Brabin, L. Interactions of the female hormonal environment, susceptibility to viral infections, and disease progression. *AIDS Patient Care and STDs*. 2002; 16(5): 211-221.

24. Labrada, L., Liang, X. H. *et al*. Age-dependent resistance to lethal alphavirus encephalitis in mice: analysis of gene expression in the central nervous system and identification of a novel interferon-inducible protective gene, mouse *ISG12*. *J Virol*. 2002; 76: 11688 - 11703.

25. Grifin, D. E., Levine, B. *et al*. Age-dependant susceptibility to fatal encephalitis - alphavirus infection of neurons. *Arch Virol*. 1994; 9: 31- 39.

26. Sigel, M. M. Influence of age on susceptibility to virus infections with particular reference to laboratory animals. *Annu Rev Microbiol*. 1952; 6: 247 - 280.

27. Blankson, A., Wiredu, E. K. *et al*. Hepatitis B and C viruses in cirrhosis of the liver in Accra, Ghana. *Ghana Med Journal*. 2005; 39(4): 132-137.

28. Acheampong, J. W. The prevalence of hepatitis B surface antigen among blood donors and jaundiced patients at Komfo Anokye Teaching Hospital, *Ghana. Med J*. 1991; 25: 313-317.

29. Emmerich, P., Thome-Bolduan, C. et al. Reverse ELISA for IgG and IgM antibodies to detect Lassa virus infections in Africa. *J Clin Virol*. 2006; (37) 4: 277 – 281.

30. World Health Organization. The yellow fever situation in Africa and South America in 2004. *Wkly Epidemiol Rec.* 2005; 80: 250-256.

31. Agadzi, V. K., Boatin, B. K. *et al.* Yellow fever in Ghana, 1977-80. *Bull WHO* 1984; 62(4): 577-583.

32. World Health Organization. *Global Alert and Response (GAR). Yellow fever.* (Accessed 15 Jan 2013). Available at: http://www.who.int/csr/don/archive/disease/yellow_fever/en/.

33. Ghana Health Service. *Annual Report, 2011. Disease surveillance; viral hepatitis.* Available at: www.ghanahealthservice.org/.../GHS%202011%20Annual%20Report%2.

# Chapter 20
## Rotavirus Diarrhoea in Ghana: From Baseline Information to Vaccine Introduction

*George E. Armah*

## Introduction

Although diarrhoeal disease can be prevented and treated, it continues to be a major cause of morbidity and mortality in children less than 5 years of age with a great majority of these being in developing countries. It is estimated that there were 1,236,000 deaths attributable to diarrhoeal disease in children in 2008. Diarrhoeal diseases are responsible for 12% of deaths in children in Africa and 11% in Asia.[1] Children between the ages of 1 month and one year carried the greatest risk (65.4%) of dying from diarrhoea.[1] The majority of mortality related to diarrhoea occurred in developing countries and eight of the ten countries responsible for 90% of all diarrhoea deaths in children globally are in Africa.[1]

The immediate causes of diarrhoea are often due to the infestation of an infectious material which includes viruses, parasites and bacteria.[2] Amongst the common bacteria pathogens of disease are diarrhoeic strains of *Escherichiacoli* which includes enteropathogenic *E.coli* (EPEC), enteroinvasive *E. coli* (EIEC), enterohemorrhagic *E. coli* (EHEC) and enterotoxigenic *E. coli* (ETEC). Whilst EPEC is the most important bacteria cause of infantile diarrhoea, EPEC is recognized as the most common cause of diarrhoea in adults.[2] Other parasites implicated in causing diarrhoea include *Entamoeba histolica*, *Giardia lamblia* and *Cryptosporidium parvum* and most of these infections are usually associated with bloody or invasive diarrhoea.[2] Viral diarrhoea in children is usually associated with a life-threatening disease, with watery diarrhoea, vomiting and fever being the most common symptoms. The major etiological agents of viral diarrhoea are rotaviruses, noroviruses, adenoviruses and astroviruses. Of these, rotaviruses have been recognized as the major cause of viral diarrhoea, responsible for 60% of all viral causes of diarrhoea in children worldwide.[3] Rotaviruses are responsible for 452,000 deaths in children globally with over 90% (420,000) of these deaths occurring in Africa and Asia.[4] Whilst improved sanitation and hygiene and increased access to safe drinking water over the last decade have reduced significantly the burden of diarrhoea diseases, there has been no dramatic effect on rotavirus infection and it continues to be a major cause of diarrhoea in children, with more than 600 associated deaths in Africa each day.[4] Studies have shown that every child in the developing world will have more than four episodes of rotavirus infection before his/her third birthday. However, only the first episode of rotavirus infection is severe and life-threatening, whereas subsequent ones are mild.[5] This observation over the past 20 years spurred the development of rotavirus vaccines as an intervention for diarrhoea due to rotavirus infection.

# Approach

## Rotavirus research at Noguchi Memorial Institute for Medical Research

The importance of rotaviruses in diarrhoea in children, although well established in the developed world, was grossly underestimated in Africa because of the lack of expertise and cost of its diagnosis. During the period 1970 to 1990, rotavirus detection was mainly by electron-microscopy and by the enzyme-linked immunosorbent assay (ELISA) diagnostic method. With the availability of a commercial ELISA kit in the 1990s, the way was paved for an in-depth look at the role played by rotaviruses in diarrhoea in children. With the availability of these two diagnostic tools in the Department, the initial research thrust was therefore focused on providing baseline data on the natural history and the prevalence of rotavirus infection in Ghana. With the designation of the Electron Microscopy and Histopathology Department as a WHO Regional Rotavirus Reference Laboratory in 2004, the diagnostic capacity of the laboratory was further enhanced to include the genotyping of strains by molecular methods. The enhanced diagnostic capacity of the Department brought with it a change in rotavirus research. The overall objective of our research for the last two decades has been to provide evidence-based data needed to support advocacy for the recognition of rotavirus as an important cause of diarrhoea in children in Ghana and Africa. In preparation for the introduction of rotavirus vaccines in the Expanded Programme of Immunization (EPI) programme. The research thrust in the Department has thus been (i) conducting epidemiological including burden of disease studies, (ii) conducting efficacy studies on available rotavirus vaccines and (iii) providing training and leadership on rotavirus diagnosis to other African countries and advocacy for the introduction of rotavirus vaccines.

## Epidemiology and burden of disease studies

Over the last decade, an active and passive surveillance for rotavirus-associated diarrhoea was set up at sentinel sites in the Upper East and Greater Accra Regions to provide the baseline data for rotavirus infection and strain types in Ghana. Between July 1997 and August 2009, an active surveillance for rotavirus infection was carried out in the Kassena Nankana District (KND) of the Upper East Region to collect baseline data on the epidemiology of disease, seasonality of disease, risk factors and the distribution of strains.

The KND is one of the nine districts in the Upper East Region of Ghana. It is bordered by the Republic of Burkina Faso to the north, the Bolgatanga Municipality and the Bongo District to south and east, Sissala and Mamprusi West districts to the west and south west. The KND has an area of about 1,675 km$^2$ and a population of 140,000 living in roughly 13,000 dispersed compounds. It has recently been split into the Kassena Nankana East and Kassena Nankana West districts. The main occupation of the people is subsistence farming. Diarrhoea surveillance sites were set up in the health facilities and the only hospital in the District, the War Memorial Hospital (WMH) in Navrongo which is the district capital. All incidences of diarrhoea were collated and stool samples collected for testing for rotavirus shedding. In addition, demographic data, history of illness, vaccination, duration of diarrhoea, peak number of stools passed per day, duration of vomiting, peak frequency of vomiting per day, degree of fever, dehydration, severity of diarrhoea[6] and treatment outcomes were collected.

From September 2009 to date, the sentinel surveillance in KND has expanded to include the diarrhoea disease burden in children at Korle Bu Teaching Hospital (KBTH) in Accra and Komfo Anokye Teaching Hospital (KATH) in Kumasi. Additional data on the number of diarrhoea hospitalizations, proportion of diarrhoea hospitalizations attributable to rotavirus, age-specific diarrhoea hospitalizations attributable to rotaviruses and duration of hospitalization for rotavirus-associated diarrhoea were collected on admission for diarrhoea at these hospitals.

## Rotavirus detection and strain type characterization

Stool specimens were collected from children below the age of five years who sought treatment for diarrhoea at the health centres in the KND or were hospitalized with diarrhoea at the Navrongo WMH, KBTH and KATH after obtaining informed consent from their mothers and caregivers. The stool samples were tested for rotaviruses and the isolated viruses characterized using molecular methods. Diarrhoea was defined as the passage of more than three looser-than-normal stools within 24 hours. Rotavirus antigen detection in stools was carried out on 10% stool suspensions with the commercial DAKO Rotavirus ELISA kit (Rotavirus IDEIA™ Dako Diagnostic Ltd., Cambridgeshire, UK) following manufacturer's instructions.[7] Stool samples were also tested for rotaviruses using poly acrylamide gel electrophoresis (PAGE). Briefly, double stranded ribonucleic acid (dsRNA) was extracted from 10% (w/v) suspension of stool sample in phosphate buffered saline (0.01 M PBS pH 7.2) prepared and purified as previously reported.[8] The purified dsRNA was electrophoresed in a discontinuous gel buffer system on a 12% poly acrylamide gel for 18 hours[7] followed by silver staining.[9]

The genotypes of isolated rotavirus strains were determined by reverse transcription polymerase chain reaction (RT-PCR). Briefly, viral

RNA was extracted from 10% faecal suspensions in PBS and purified using the RNaid Kit (BIO 101, Southern Cross Biotechnology, USA). The purified RNA was reverse transcribed and amplified after specific priming with either VP7 or VP4 consensus primer pairs. The cDNA generated was then used for G and P typing with G and P specific oligonucleotide primers (Table 20.1 (a, b)) as previously described.[10,11] The amplified gene products were examined by gel electrophoresis in 1.2% agarose and the genotypes assigned accordingly based on the sizes of the amplicons.

## Vaccine efficacy studies

Historically, whilst rotavirus vaccines have shown good efficacy in the United States and other developed countries, they showed little, varying or no efficacy in developing countries. Earlier trials of first-generation rotavirus vaccines in the Central African Republic, Rwanda, The Gambia, and Peru showed little or no efficacy in contrast to the high efficacy shown in other developed countries.[12] Given the history of rotavirus vaccine performance in the developing world, the World Health Organization (WHO) Expert Committee on Biological Standardization recommended that the efficacy of "new" rotavirus vaccines should be demonstrated in diverse geographical regions including developing countries before their widespread implementation.

A grant from the Programme for Appropriate Technology in Health (PATH) as part of a multi-site (three sites in Africa: Kenya, Mali and Ghana) to conduct a randomized, double-blind (and in-house blind), placebo-controlled trial to evaluate the efficacy, safety and immunogenicity of RotaTeq™ among infants.[13] Approximately 2,200 infants were randomly assigned to 1 of 2 treatment groups (1 RotaTeq™: 1 placebo) to receive three (3) oral doses of RotaTeq™/placebo at 6, 10 and 14 weeks of age in Navrongo, Ghana. The primary objective was to evaluate the efficacy of a 3-dose regimen of RotaTeq™ against severe (as measured by Vesikari Clinical Scoring System ≥11) rotavirus gastroenteritis caused by any rotavirus serotype occurring at least 14 days following the third dose in each region (i.e. Asia and Africa). All participants were followed after vaccination and all serious adverse events (SAEs) occurring within 14 days following each dose and deaths, or vaccine-related SAEs occurring at any time during the study was documented.

# Findings and discussion

## Epidemiology and burden of disease studies

A total of 2,086 diarrhoea episodes were identified of which 843 (39%) were shedding rotavirus. Twenty-four percent of children shedding rotaviruses were aged less than 6 months, 64 % of infants under 12 months of age and 88% of children under 18 months of age (Table 20.2). It was, however, not common in children older than 36 months. The greatest period of risk was 6-18 months and rotavirus-positive diarrhoea episodes tended to be more acute, causing vomiting and greater dehydration and more likely to require hospitalization. More than 60% of hospitalized children with diarrhoea were found to be excreting rotaviruses in their stools. Rotavirus infection was seasonal, with peak infection occurring during the cool dry months of October to April (Fig. 20.1). Risk factors for rotavirus included between 6 to 18 months of age wasting, high Vesikari score and the episode occurring in the dry season.

Rotavirus strains bearing the VP7 genotypes G1 and G2 consti-tuted more than 65% of all G types detected between 2007 and 2010 in Ghana. The genotypes G2P[6], G3P[4] and G1P[8] made up more than 50% of genotypes detected in hospitalized children (Table 20.2). There was a high diversity of viruses and the dominant strain types changed from year to year as shown in Fig.20.3. The unusual strain types G1P[6] G3[p6] and G1P[4] were also commonly detected. In 2009 and 2010, G10 and G12 strains, which are common in cattle, were also detected for the first time in the human population in Ghana.

Table 20.1(a):    VP7 GENOTYPING PRIMERS

| Primer | Sequence (5'-3') | Position (nt) | Strain (genotype) |
|---|---|---|---|
| Gouvea/Itturiza-Gomara/Banerjee Primers | | | |
| Beg9 | GGCTTTAAAAGAGA-GAATTTCCGTCTGG | 1-28 | 5' |
| End9 | GGTACACATCATACAAT-TCTAATCTAAG | 1062-1036 | 3' |
| RVG9 | GGTACATCATACAATTCT | 1062-1044 | 3' |
| aAT8 | GTCACACCATTTG-TAAATTCG | 178-198 | 69M (G8) 885 bp |
| aBT1 | CAAGTACTCAAATCAAT-GATGG | 314-335 | Wa (G1) 749 bp |
| aCT2 | CAATGATATTAACACATTT-TCTGTG | 411-435 | DS-1 (G2) 652 bp |
| aDT4 | CGTTTCTGGTGAG-GAGTTG | 480-498 | ST-3 (G4) 583 bp |
| aET3 | CGTTTGAAGAAGTT-GCAACAG | 689-709 | P (G3) 374 bp |
| aFT9 | CTAGATGTAACTA-CAACTAC | 757-776 | W161 (G9) 306 bp |
| G10 | ATGTCAGACTACARA-TACTGG | 666-687 | (G10) 397 bp |
| G12 | CCGATGGACG-TAACGTTGTA | 548-567 | (G12) 515 bp |
| DAS/ Cunliffe Primers | | | |
| 9Con1 | TAGCTCCTTTTAATG-TATGG | 37-56 | 5' + sense |
| 9Con2 | GTATAA AATACTTGCCACCA | 922-941 | 3' |
| 9T1-1 | TCTTGTCAAAG-CAAATAATG | 176-195 | Wa (G1) 158 bp |
| 9T1-2 | GTTAGAAATGAT-TCTCCACT | 262-281 | S2 (G2) 244 bp |

Table 20.1(a):    VP7 GENOTYPING PRIMERS (continued)

| Primer | Sequence (5'-3') | Position (nt) | Strain (genotype) |
|---|---|---|---|
| Gouvea/Itturiza-Gomara/Banerjee Primers | | | |
| 9T-3P | GTCCAGTTGCAGT-GTTAGC | 484-503 | 107E1B (G3) 466 bp |
| 9T-4 | GGGTCGATGGAAAATTCT | 423-440 | ST3 (G4) 403 bp |
| 9T-9B | TATAAAGTCCATTGCAC | 131-147 | 116E (G9) 110 bp |
| MW-8 | TCTTCAAAAGTCGTAGTG | 670-688 | MW (G8) 651 bp |
| Rotavirus VP7 Animal Primer Set | | | |
| sBeg9 | GGCTTTAAAAGAGA-GAATTTC | 1-21 | 5' |
| aFT5 | GACGTAACAACGAG-TACATG | 779-760 | OSU G5 |
| aDT6 | GATTCTACACAG-GAACTAG | 499-481 | UK G6 |
| aHT8 | GTGTCTAATCCGGAACCG | 273-256 | B37 G8 |
| aET10 | GAAGTCGCAACGGCTGAA | 714-697 | B223 G10 |
| aBT1 | GCAACTCAGATTGCT-GATGAC | 336-316 | YM G11 |

Table20.1(b):    VP4 GENOTYPING PRIMERS

| Primer | Human-Sequence (5'-3') | Position (nt) | Strain/ Genotype |
|---|---|---|---|
| Con2 | ATTTCGGACCATT-TATAACC | 868-887 | 3' |
| Con3 | TGGCTTCGCTCATT-TATAGACA | 11-32 | 5' |
| 1-T1 | TCT ACT TGG ATA ACG TGC | 336-356 | KU P[8] |
| 1-T1VN | CGT GCA GCT AGG TCA TCT | 336-356 | Vietnam P[8] |
| 1-T1Wa | CGT GCA ATT GGG TCA TCT | 336-356 | Jrg P[8] |

Table20.1(b):    VP4 GENOTYPING PRIMERS (continued)

| Primer | Human-Sequence (5'-3') | Position (nt) | Strain/ Genotype |
|---|---|---|---|
| 2T-1 | CTATTGTTAGAGGTTA-GAGTC | 474-494 | RV5 P[4] |
| 3T-1 | TGTTGATTAGTT-GGATTCAA | 259-278 | 1076 P[6] |
| 4T-1 | TGAGACAT-GCAATTGGAC | 385-402 | K8 P[9] |
| 5T-1 | ATCATAGTTAGTAGTCGG | 575-594 | 69M P[10] |
| Animal-Sequence (5'-3') | | | |
| pGott | GCTTCAACGTCCTT-TAACATCAG | 465-487 423 bp | Gottfried P[7] |
| pOSU | CTTTATCGGTGGA-GAATACGTCAC | 389-412 502 bp | OSU P[7] |
| Puk | GCCAGGTGTCGCAT-CAGAG | 336-354 555 bp | UK P[5] |
| pNCDV | CGAACGCGGGGGTGG-TAGTTG | 269-289 | NCDV P[1] |
| pB223 | GGAACGTATTCTAATC-CGGTG | 574-594 314 bp | B223 P[11] |

Table 20.2:    Age-Specific Incidence of Rotavirus Infection in Ghanaian Children Hospitalized with Diarrhoea (2007-2009)

| Age Group (months) | Number Tested | Rotavirus +ve (%) |
|---|---|---|
| <1 | 28 | 10 (35.7) |
| 2-6 | 525 | 191 (36.3) |
| 7-12 | 835 | 337 (40.4) |
| 13-18 | 491 | 206 (42.0) |
| 19-24 | 207 | 90 (43.5) |
| >36 | 58 | 9(15.5) |
| All | 2086 | 39.3 |

Table 20.3: Distribution of rotavirus G and P genotypes among children <5 years of age in Ghana (2007– 2007)

| P- Type | Gl | G2 | G3 | G4 | GS | G9 | GlO | G12 | Gnt |
|---------|----|----|----|----|----|----|-----|-----|-----|
| P[4] | 23 | 71 | 2 | 7 | 1 | 0 | 1 | 0 | 8 |
| P[6] | 67 | 57 | 61 | 7 | 0 | 16 | 26 | 1 | 16 |
| P[B] | 247 | 21 | 5 | 2 | 0 | 4 | 1 | 1 | 12 |
| P[nt] | 33 | 3 | 2 | 0 | 0 | 0 | 1 | 0 | 10 |
| All | 370 | 152 | 70 | 16 | 1 | 20 | 29 | 2 | 46 |

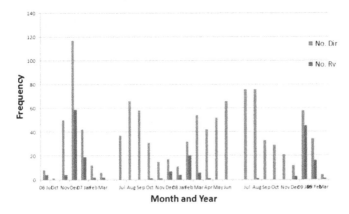

Fig.20.1 Seasonality of RV Incidence in Ghana (2006-2009)

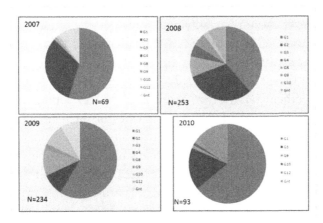

Fig.20.2 Circulating Rotavirus Genotypes in Ghana (2007-2009)

# Vaccine efficacy studies

Out of a total of 5,468 (98.3%) subjects enrolled across the three sites in Africa, 2,200 subjects were enrolled and randomized in Ghana to receive either the RotaTeq™ rotavirus vaccine (n=1098) or placebo (n=1102). More than 95% of the subjects received all 3 doses of the RotaTeq™ vaccine (n=1054) or placebo (n=1047). The results of the efficacy analysis have been recently reported.[13] The mean age of participants on enrolment was 58.8 days and there were similar numbers of males and females enrolled. More than 78% of the children who received the vaccine responded and had >3 fold rise in anti-rotavirus specific serum IgA.[14] The efficacy of the vaccine against severe rotavirus diarrhoea in Ghanaian children during the first and second year of follow-up post-immunization was 65.1% (CI 35.5, 81.9) and 29.4% (CI -64.6, 20.7) respectively. The efficacy against severe rotavirus-associated diarrhoea during the entire two years of follow up was 55.5% (CI 28.0, 73.1). The vaccine was safe in Ghanaian children, with only 1.4% and 1.3% of participants in the vaccine and placebo arms respectively reporting of any adverse event, which were mainly infestations and infections.

Studies in the Department over the years have helped to delineate the important role played by rotaviruses in diarrhoea in children and its large burden of disease. It has also brought to light the vast diversity of strains circulating in the country and the continuing annual shift in strain dominance. It is gratifying to note that the findings of these studies provided the evidence-based data that the Ghana Ministry of Health needed to take a decision on the introduction of rotavirus vaccines in Ghana in June 2012. The decision has informed and influenced other countries in Africa and the developing world to consider the inclusion of rotavirus vaccines in their EPI programs. The Department will continue to evaluate these vaccines and monitor the circulating genotypes as the vaccine roll out and the coverage increases. Our work on rotavirus diarrhoea and the contribution to the advocacy for the introduction of rotavirus vaccines in the EPI will aid in preventing a large proportion of the over 2000 annual rotavirus-associated diarrhoea deaths in Ghanaian children (>3% of the estimated under-five mortality of 57,000) from dying from this vaccine-preventable disease and also help to reduce significantly severe diarrhoea hospitalizations, mainly caused by this virus in Ghanaian children.

# Acknowledgements

We will like to thank all parents who consented to letting their children take part in the studies, staff of the EM/Histopathology Department of the Noguchi Institute and the Rotavirus teams at the Navrongo Health Research Centre and the Paediatric Department of the Korle Bu Teaching Hospital for their contribution to the successful conduct of this study. We thank also our sponsors, the Gates Foundation, WHO, MERCK and PATH for all their support.

# Reference

1.  Lui, L., Johnson, H. L., Cousens, S. *et al*. Global, regional, and national causes of child mortality: an updated systematic analysis for 2010 with time trends since 2000. *The Lancet*. 2012; 379 (9832): 2051-2161

2.  Schorling, J. B., Wanke, C. A., Schorling, S. K., McAuliffe, J. F., de Souza, M. A., Guerrant, R. L. A prospective study of persistent diarrhoea among children in an urban Brazilian slum:patterns of occurrence and etiologic agents. *Am J Epidemiol*. 1990;132(1):144-156

3.  Iturriza-Gomara, M., Desselberger, U., and Gray ,J. Molecular Epidemiology of Rotaviruses: Genetic Mechanisms Associated with diversity. In: Desselberger, U. and Gray, J. eds. Amsterdam: Elsevier. 2003:317-344.

4.  Tate, J. E., Burton, A. H., Boschi-Pinto, C. *et al*. 2008 estimates of worldwide rotavirus-associated mortality in children younger than 5 years before the introduction of universal rotavirusvaccination programme: a systematic review and meta-analysis. *The Lancet Infect Dis*. 2012; 12(2): 136-141

5.  Parasher, U. D., Breese, J., Gentsch J. Rotavirus. *Emerg Infect Dis*. 1998; 4: 561-570

6.  Ruuska, T., Vesikari, T. Rotavirus disease in Finnish children: use of numerical scores for clinical severity of diarrhoeal episodes. *Scand J Infect Dis.* 1990; 22:259-267.

7.  Armah, G. E., Steele, A. D., Binka, F. N. *et al.* Changing patterns of rotavirus genotypes in Ghana: emergence of human rotavirus G9 as a major cause of diarrhoea in children. *J Clin Microbiol.* 2003; 41:2317-2322.

8.  Laemmli, U. K. Cleavage of structural proteins during the assembly of the head of bacteriophage T4. *Nature.*1970; 227(5259): 680 - 685.

9.  Herring, A. J., Inglis, N. F., Ojeh, C. K., Snodgrass, D. R. and Menzies, J. D. Rapid diagnosis of rotavirus infection by direct detection of viral nucleic acid in silver-stained polyacrylamide gels. *J Clin Microbiol.* 1982; 16(3): 473 – 477

10. Gentsch, J. R., Glass, R. I., Woods, P., Gouvea, V., Gorziglia, M., Flores, J., Das, B. K. and Bhan, M. K. Identification of group A rotavirus gene 4 types by polymerase chain reaction. *J Clin Microbiol.* 1992; 30(6): 1365 - 1373.

11. Gouvea, V., Glass, R. I., Woods, P., Taniguchi, K., Clark, H. F., Forrester, B. and Fang, Z. Y. Polymerase chain reaction amplification and typing of rotavirus nucleic acid from stool specimens. *J Clin Microbiol.* 1990; 28(2): 276 - 282.

12. Georges-Courbot, M. C., Monges, J., Siopathis, M. R. *et al.* Evaluation of the efficacy of a low-passage bovine rotavirus (strain WC3) vaccine in children in Central Africa. *Res Virol.* 1991; 142:405-411.

13. Armah, G. E., Sow, S. O., Breiman, R. F. *et al.* Efficacy of pentavalent rotavirus vaccine against severe rotavirus gastroenteritis in infants in developing countries in sub-Saharan Africa: a randomised, double-blind, placebo-controlled trial. *Lancet.* 2010; 376:606-614.

14. Armah, G. E., Breiman, R. F., Milagritos, D. T., Samba, S. S., Dallas, M. J., Steele, A. D., Binka, F., Ojwando, J., Ciarlet, M. and Neuzil, K. M. Immunogenicity of the pentavalent rotavirus vaccine in African infants. *Vaccine.* 2012; 30 Suppl 1: A86-93.

# Chapter 21
# Phytomedicines: Safety and Efficacy Studies on Ghanaian Medicinal Plants

*Regina Appiah-Opong, Nii-Ayi Ankrah, Alexander K. Nyarko and Mark Ofosuhene*

## Introduction

Phytomedicine, the use of plants or plant parts to treat various ailments, remains one of the forms of treatments used by a large part of the world's population. According to the World Health Organization (WHO), about 70-80% of the world's population, especially those living in developing countries, depends on plant medicines either in part or entirely.[1] Various reasons have been given for the use of plant medicines, and these include inadequate orthodox health care facilities, especially in the rural areas, limited financial access to health services; cheaper alternative to orthodox medicines, anecdotal evidence of successful treatments with plant medicines and the strong link between the culture of populations and medicine.

A wide range of conventional drugs has originally been derived from plants. An analysis of the origin of the drugs revealed that at the dawn of the twenty-first century, 11% of the 252 drugs considered as basic and essential by the WHO were exclusively of flowering plant origin.[2] The most significant impact of plant-derived drugs was probably experienced in the area of anticancer. The discovery of vinblastine, vincristine (from *Catharanthus roseus* L.), taxol (from *Taxus brevifolia* Nutt.) and camptothecin (*Camptotheca acuminate* Decne) has improved the chemotherapy used against cancers.[3]

In Ghana, traditional medicine practitioners (TMPs) produce most of the plant medicines on the market. The mention of medicinal plants use usually raises intense debates between TMPs and orthodox medicine practitioners (OMPs). However, the significant role of each of these practitioners in the management of various diseases is well known. Africa is naturally endowed with numerous medicinal plants, but a majority of plant-derived drugs have not yet been explored or discovered. Obviously, development of natural products such as plant medicines to drugs is time consuming, difficult and capital intensive. Therefore, the joint effort of TMPs and OMPs will be useful in bringing together plant medicines and conventional medical practice for the benefit of the public.

The widely held belief of lay people is that "natural" can be equated to "safe".[4] In USA, interactions of herbal medicines with synthetic ones have become of particular interest. Between 1999 and 2002, more than 50 papers were published on interactions between St John's wort and prescribed drugs only.[5,6,7] The consequences of herb-drug interactions can be: (a) beneficial effects, such as cancer prevention; (b) undesirable effects; such as alteration of pharmacological effects of co-administered drugs; (c) harmful effects, such as organ toxicity or carcinogenesis.[8,9] The interaction may be due to either induction or inhibition of drug metabolizing enzymes (particularly cytochrome P450 enzymes). The result is either a decrease or an increase in the action of the administered orthodox drug, thus altering the treatment outcome.

Scientists at the Noguchi Memorial Institute for Medical Research (NMIMR) have conducted research on the efficacy of a number of plant medicines used for the treatment or management of diseases such as diabetes mellitus, hypertension, asthma and HIV/AIDS in Ghana. Toxicity studies on most of these plant medicines have also been conducted and reported.

# Approach

### Anti-diabetes studies

Diabetic mice and volnteers were treated with plant extracts for 13 and 12 weeks, respectively. Blood samples were collected and changes in fasting plasma glucose levels were measured spectrophotometrically.[10,11]

## Anti-asthmatic studies

*Thonningia sanguinea* and *Parquetina nigrescens* extracts and fractions were tested for their anti-anaphylactic properties.[12,13] Guinea pigs were sensitized using crystalline egg albumin treatment schedules with plant extracts were followed throughout the sensitization period of 28 days. Anaphylactic contractions in a piece of ileum (obtained from a sacrificed guinea pig) elicited by the addition of antigen was recorded with a transducer. Inhibitory activity towards blood phospholipase $A_2$ was also determined.

## Anti-HIV studies

To determine the *in vitro* anti-HIV activity of *Ocimum gratissimum* (GHX-2), *Ficus polita* (GHX-6), *Clausena anisata* (GHX-7), *Alchornea cordifolia* (GHX-26) and *Elaeophorbia drupifera* cultured human cell line infected with the HIV-1 strain $HTLVIII_B$ were treated with the plant extracts.[14] The modified tetrazolium-based colorimetric (MTT) assay and HIV reverse transcriptase (RT) assay.[14,15] were used to determine the susceptibility of the HIV virus to the plant extracts. Inhibition of Molt-4 and Molt-4/HIV cell replication by selected plant extracts was assessed using the Trypan blue exclusion method. Cells were counted, treated with extracts and re-counted two and four days respectively after treatment. In addition, uninfected Molt-4–Molt-4/ HIVco cultures were cultured in the presence of plant extracts and AZT. After incubation the cultures were examined for HIV-1 cytopathic effect (CPE). The effect of the plant extracts on HIV proviral DNA copying (HIV proviral DNA-dependent synthesis by taq polymerase) was studied using polymerase chain reaction (PCR).[16]

# Findings and Discussion

## Anti-diabetes studies

Diabetes mellitus is an endocrine disease caused by either absolute or relative deficiency of insulin, a hormone that helps to remove glucose from the blood. Insulin deficiency causes elevation in levels of glucose in the blood and urine, known as hyperglycaemia and glucosuria, respectively. The two major types of diabetes mellitus are type 1, characterized by absolute lack of insulin, and type 2 which is due to a relative lack of insulin or inability to utilize it.[17] In type I diabetes, the rise in blood glucose level is due to destruction of β-cells that produce insulin. Thus, it is known as insulin-dependent diabetes since the patients depend on insulin treatment. It is commonly detected in people under 30 years of age. On the other hand, with type II diabetes ,the rise in blood glucose levels is due to lack of insulin production, insufficient insulin action (resistant cell), which results in the failure of β-cells to produce insulin. This condition is commonly detected in people above 40 years. Complications associated with both type I and II diabetes include stroke, heart attack, kidney disease, eye disease and damage of the nerves. Some Ghanaians manage the disease with plant medicines.

An aqueous extract of this plant was used at the CSRPM at Akuapem Mampong to manage diabetes mellitus. It was observed that when administered orally to diabetic patients for two weeks, the extract decreased blood glucose levels, although not to normal levels (Table 21.1).[18] Interestingly, the extract did not alter glucose levels in healthy non-diabetic humans.[10,18] Subsequently, the researchers have shown that *I. arrecta* extract promotes insulin release and is therefore not effective in animals whose pancreases have been destroyed.[19,20,21]

These studies demonstrate that *I. arrecta* extract is largely safe but would not be useful for the management of severe diabetes mellitus because of its inability to bring blood glucose to normal levels. The extract would also not be useful for type 1 diabetes because of its dependence on an intact and functional pancreas. Since *I. arrecta* is currently being used at the CSRPM to manage diabetes mellitus, it will be worthwhile to conduct further studies to determine the efficacy of this extract on mild cases of the disease.

Investigations were also conducted on *Ocimum canum*, known as 'ɛme' in Akan or '*ahamɛ*' in Ewe, also used to manage diabetes mellitus. Extracts of this medicinal plant cause decreases in fasting blood glucose levels and body weight in both diabetic and non-diabetic animals.[22] The change in fasting blood glucose levels in extract-treated animals was -60%, whereas only a change of -12% was observed in control animals. The plant extract also enhanced insulin release in a concentration-dependent manner. Interestingly, *O. canum* extract decreases total cholesterol levels and low-density lipoprotein (LDL), known as "bad cholesterol" levels, which is a risk factor for heart disease. On the other hand, the extract increased levels of high-density lipoprotein (HDL), known as "good cholesterol" which protects against heart disease.[11] Therefore, *O. canum* extract, in addition to controlling blood glucose, may decrease a diabetic patient's risk of heart disease.

The NMIMR, in collaboration with the Department of Biochemistry, University of Ghana, investigated another herbal medicine used by some Ghanaian diabetic patients to manage diabetes mellitus known as ADD-199. It is prepared from *Maytenus senegalensis*, *Annona senegalensis*, *Kigelia africana* and *Lannea welwitschii*. A daily dose of 100mg/kg body weight effectively lowered streptozotocin (STZ)-induced hypergycaemia in mice.[23] Phytochemical analysis showed that ADD-199 contains among other things, alkaloids, terpenoids, tannins and flavonoids. The hypoglycemic activity was associated with the alkaloidal content.

Table 21.1:   Effect of *I. arrecta* extract on fasting blood glucose levels of diabetic patients

| Patient No. | Fasting plasma glucose levels (mmol/L) | | | |
|---|---|---|---|---|
| | Wk 0 | Wk 4 | Wk 8 | Wk 12 |
| 1 | 11.5 | 10.0 | 10.2 | nd |
| 2 | 10.4 | 9.2 | 8.4 | nd |
| 3 | 8.0 | 7.0 | 7.2 | 7.5 |
| 4 | 13.6 | 10.5 | 9.2 | 11.0 |
| 5 | 9.0 | 7.5 | 7.4 | 7.2 |
| 6 | 13.2 | 10.3 | 10.1 | 10.4 |

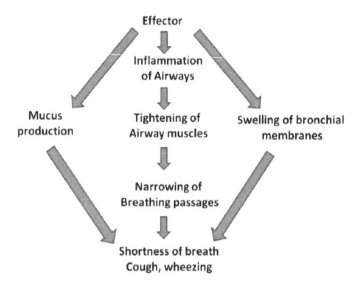

*Figure 21.1: A model of immunopathology of asthma (Adapted from Coffey and Peters-Golden, 2003).*

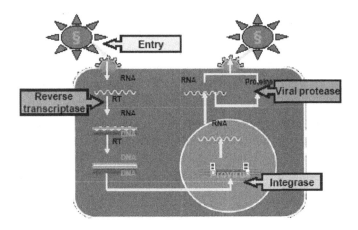

*Figure 21. 2: Life cycle of human immunodeficiency virus (Adapted from www.medscape.com).*

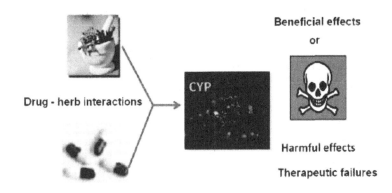

*Figure 21. 3: Herb-drug interactions mediated by cytochrome P450.*

## Anti-asthmatic studies

Asthma is a health condition that affects the airways, resulting in difficulty in breathing. It is characterized by abrupt, often violent, and recurrent reversible airway obstruction. Generally, asthmatics have a respiratory disorder in which the body becomes hypersensitive or allergic to specific substances called allergens or antigens. In allergic persons, subsequent exposure to the specific allergen causes an abnormal reaction called anaphylaxis that involves cell damage and release of pro-inflammatory chemical substances such as histamine and pro-inflammatory eicosanoids that contract smooth muscles and thus precipitate the characteristic symptoms of asthma, which is mainly difficulty in breathing.[24,25,26] Figure 21.1 shows a model of immunopathology of asthma.[26]

Addy and Nyarko performed anaphylaxis experiments using a guinea pig as a model to investigate how two Ghanaian plant medicines prepared from *Thonningia sanguinea* and *Parquetina nigrescens* known as *Kwabedwaa* in Akan or *Ahlɔɛmadui* in Ewe and *abakamo* in Akan, respectively affect some of the biochemical processes involved in asthma.[27] Extract treated group showed 30% anaphylactic contractions at 100μg/ml antigen concentrations, whilst the control experiment showed 78% contractions. The investigations revealed that *Thonningia sanguinea* extract inhibits guinea pig smooth muscle contractions in response to an antigen. It also reduces the sensitivity of smooth muscles to contractile agents such as histamine. Furthermore, the extract decreases lung content and the release of pro-inflammatory eicosanoids that contract smooth muscles. Extract-treated muscles exhibited 17nmol/ml/min Phospholipase A (PLA) activity compared to the control that showed a higher activity of 27nm/ml/min. The *P. nigrescens* extract, in particular, inhibited the activity of blood phospholipase $A_2$ (sPLA2), an enzyme that mobilizes arachidonic acid from membranes for the synthesis of eicosanoids.[12,13]

## Anti-HIV studies

The human immunodeficiency virus (HIV) infection causes acquired immune deficiency syndrome (AIDS) which is characterized by progressive loss of CD4+ helper cells of T lymphocytes. As a result there is severe immunosuppression and opportunistic infections that rarely occur when the immune function is intact. Figure 21.2 shows the life cycle of HIV. Two distinct species of HIV (HIV-1 and HIV-2) have been identified. Nearly 40 million adults and children worldwide live with HIV.

Active and progressive HIV infections may be acute or chronic in nature. In the case of the latter, infected cells live far longer than the former, and serve as sources for virus production, whilst latently infected cells are reservoirs.[28] Several nucleoside analogs including 3-azido-2', 3'-dideoxythymidine (AZT) have been developed to inhibit virus production and cytopathicity in acutely infected cells.[29] The nucleoside analogs act by inhibiting HIV-specified reverse transcriptase (RT).[30] Challenges to treatment of HIV infection include poor water solubility of early drugs, poor bioavailability of drugs and drug resistance.[31,32,33] Thus, it is crucial that the search for new drugs with better pharmacological properties continues.

Researchers at NMIMR performed comparative *in vitro* studies on the effects of AZT and aqueous extracts of *Ocimum gratissimum* (GHX-2), *Ficus polita* (GHX-6), *Clausena anisata* (GHX-7), *Alchornea cordifolia* (GHX-26) and *Elaeophorbia drupifera* (GHX-27) against HIV-1 and HIV-2 replication and cytopathicity.[14] All the plant extracts inhibited HIV-1 strain HTLVIII$_B$ cytopathicity (i.e. changes in cells due to HIV infection), with the leaves of GHX-2 and the seeds of GHX-26 having higher antiviral indices (110 and 90, respectively). The extracts also strongly prevented the growth of HIV-2 strain GH1. However, extract GHX-7 showed only moderate activity towards the GH1 strain whereas GHX-26 showed no activity. When treatment was delayed for two hours the plant extracts, like AZT, were still very effective against HIV-2. The plant extracts strongly inhibited HIV-1 reverse transcriptase activity. The HIV-1 proviral DNA copying as determined in a polymerase chain reaction was completely blocked by GHX-2 and GHX-6, whilst GHX-26 and GHX-27 showed very moderate inhibitory activity.

The study has shown that the aqueous plant extracts were effective inhibitors of HIV-1 and HIV-2 replication. Early fusion of chronically infected HIV cells with uninfected cells was not affected by AZT, but it was inhibited by GHX-2, GHX-6, GHX-26 and GHX-27. Significantly, an extract of *E. drupifera* (GHX-27) has been identified to be selectively toxic to chronically infected cells at concentrations that are not cytotoxic to uninfected cells.

The effects of *Ocimum gratissimum* (GHX-2), *Ficus polita* (GHX-6), *Clausena anisata* (GHX-7), *Alchornea cordifolia* (GHX-26), *Elaeophorbia drupifera* (GHX-27), and AZT on *in vitro* HIV-1 and HIV-2 replication and cytopathicity were also compared.

## 4. Herb-drug interactions

Natural products such as foods and herbal products may potentially cause harmful effects when taken together with drugs. Concomitant intake of herbal products and allopathic medicines increases the possibility of herb-drug interactions (Figure 21.3). The effect of a particular herbal product on the efficacy and/or toxicity of another drug, referred to as herb-drug interaction, is an important issue in healthcare that warrants consideration. Like drug-drug interactions herb-drug interactions contsitute a phenomenon that can evade regulatory agencies. Herbal medicines are usually mixtures of more than one active ingredient, therefore the likelihood of herbal interaction is theoretically higher than drug-drug interaction. Herb-drug interactions are a major concern, especially due to the potential of adverse effects. Herbal products may modulate important drug metabolizing enzymes such as cytochrome P450s (CYPs). Herbal medicines such as St. John's wort, ginseng and gingko, which are freely available over the counter, have been reported to cause serious clinical interactions when co-administered with prescribed medicines for treatment of heart diseases, cancers and HIV/AIDS among others.[34] St. John's wort, which is commonly used as an anti-depressant, has been implicated in a potentially fatal interaction with cyclosporine.

Several known pharmacokinetic drug interactions are associated with phase I bio-transformation enzymes, particularly CYP enzymes. Pharmacokinetic CYP-mediated drug interactions, one of the major causes of attrition in drug development, involves induction and inhibition of the CYP enzymes, with the latter being more common.[8,35] Enzyme induction occurs when a substance foreign to the body (drug or herbal product) stimulates the synthesis of CYP isoenzymes. On the other hand, enzyme inhibition occurs when there is a reduction in enzyme activity due to the presence of a foreign substance (inhibitor). Drug interactions involving CYPs have also been identified as important causes of adverse drug reactions and therapeutic failure.[36] Thus, inhibition of CYP enzymes could result in accumulation of drugs, and subsequently lead to clinically important drug interactions.[37] Serious toxicity may develop rapidly if the inhibited drug has a narrow therapeutic window. The observed induction and inhibition of CYP enzymes by natural products in the presence of a prescribed drug has led to the general acceptance that natural products can have adverse effects, contrary to the popular belief in their safety, especially in countries where there is an active practice of ethnomedicine.[38] Hence, it is necessary that foods and herbal products be assessed for their potential to cause harmful drug-food/herb interactions.

Thus, the researchers at NMIMR are investigating CYP enzyme-mediated drug-drug and herb-drug interactions of plant and orthodox medicines used to manage or treat infectious diseases in Ghana. These findings will indicate the drugs, and herbal medicines with the potential to cause drug interactions. It will be a useful prescription guide for medical practitioners and traditional medicine practitioners for the prevention of adverse drug interactions that involve anti-malarial, anti-tuberculosis and anti-HIV drugs, and plant remedies. The outcome will also provide useful information for combination therapy for these infectious diseases. Combination therapy is an important antidote for delaying the onset of drug resistance, as it may prolong therapeutic life and improve treatment outcome.

# Conclusion

Plant medicines are a rich source of potentially important drugs. Several clinically important drugs have already been obtained from plant sources. It is necessary that scientists investigate the world of plants with the assistance of traditional medicine practitioners to scientifically establish the safety and efficacy of plant medicines used to treat various ailments. Unfortunately, most of the investigations performed on plant medicines are not continued up to a point when useful products are developed. Scientists have attributed the abrupt termination of studies on medicinal plants to the lack of sources of funding. It is important that the government recognizes that in addition to other resources of the nation, medicinal plants form a rather significant category of resources that has not been well explored. Thus, the government must make funds available for drug discovery studies. All plant medicinal products being used by humans and commercialized must meet standards set by the WHO and the Food and Drugs Authority of Ghana. They must be tested to ensure their quality, efficacy and safety in order to safeguard human health.

# References

1.  World Health Organization. Traditional Medicine. 2008. WHO Fact Sheet 134. Available from: http://www.who.int/mediacentre/ factsheets/ fs134/en/.
2.  Rates, S. M. Plants as a source of drugs. *Toxicon*. 2001; 39: 603-613.
3.  Newman, D. J., Cragg, G. M., Snader, K. M. Natural products as sources of new drugs over the period. 1981-2002. *J Nat Prod*. 2003; 66: 1022-1037.
4.  Ernst, E. Herbal medicines – they are popular but are they also safe? Eur *J Clin Pharmacol*.2006; 62: 1-2.
5.  Hammerness, P., Basch, E., Ulbricht, C., Barrette, E.P., Foppa, I., Bent, S. et al. St John's wort: a systematic review of adverse effects and drug interactions for the consultation psychiatrist. *Psychosomatics*. 2003; 44:271-282.
6.  Henderson, L., Yue, Q. Y., Bergquist, C., Gerden, B., Arlett, P. St John's wort (Hypericum perforatum): drug interactions and clinical outcomes. *Br J Clin Pharmacol*. 2002; 54:349-356.
7.  Schulz, V. Safety of St. John's wort extract compared to synthetic anti depressants. *Phytomedicine*. 2006;13: 199-204.
8.  Mandlekar, S., Hong, J. L., Kong, A. N. Modulation of metabolic enzymes by dietary phytochemicals: a review of mechanisms underlying beneficial versus unfavorable effects. *Curr Drug Metab*. 2006; 7: 661-675.
9.  Barone, G. W., Gurley, B. J., Ketel, B. L., Lightfoot, M. L., Abul-Ezz, S. R. Drug interaction between St. John's Wort and cyclosporine. *Ann Pharmacother*. 2000; 34: 1013-1016.

10. Sittie, A. A., Nyarko, A. K. Indigofera arrecta: Safety evaluation of an anti-diabetic plant extract in non-diabetic human volunteers. *Phytother Res.* 1998;12: 52-54.

11. Nyarko, A. K., Asare-Anane, H., Ofosuhene, M., Addy, M. E., Teye, K., Addo, P.G. Aqueous extract of Ocimum canum decreases levels of fasting blood glucose and free radicals and increases anti-atherogenic lipid levels in mice. *Vascular Pharmacol.* 2003; 39: 273-279.

12. Granata, F., Balestrieri, B., Petraroli, A., Giannattasio, G., Marone, G., Trigging, M. Secretory phospholipases A2 as multivalent mediators of inflammatory and allergic disorders. *Int Arch Allergy Immunol.* 2003; 131: 153-63.

13. Nyarko, A. K., Addy, M. E. *In vitro* screening for the anti-anaphylactic agent in Thonningia sanguinea. *J Ethnopharmacol.* 1994; 41: 45-51.

14. Ayisi, N. K., Nyadedzor, C. Comparative *in vitro* effects of AZT and extracts of Ocimum gratissimum, Ficus polita, Clausena anisata, Alchornea cordifolia and Elaeophorbia drupifera against HIV-1 and HIV-2 infections. *Antiviral Res.* 2003; 58: 25-33.

15. Nakashima, H., Masuda, M., Murakami, T., Koyanagi, Y., Matsumoto, A., Fuji, N., Yamamoto, N. Anti-human immunodeficiency virus activity of a novel synthetic peptide, T22([Tyr-5,12,Lys-7]polyphemusinII): a possible inhibitor of virus–cell fusion. *Antimicrob Agents Chemother.* 1992; 36: 1249–1255.

16. Ayisi, N. K. Differential cytopathicity and susceptibility of Ghanaian highly divergent HIV-2[GH2], prototype HIV-2[GH1], and prototype HIV-1[GH3] to inhibition by ddCyd and an dddIno. *East Afr Med J.* 1995; 72: 654–657.

17. Amoah, A. G., Owusu, S. K., Adjei, S. Diabetes in Ghana: a community based prevalence study in Greater Accra. *Diabetes Res Clin Pract.* 2002; 56: 197-205.

18. Addy, M. E., Nyarko, A. K. Diabetic patients' response to aqueous extracts of Indigofera arrecta. *Phytother Res.* 1988; 2: 192-195.

19. Addy, M. E., Addo, P., Nyarko, A. K. Indigofera arrecta prevents the development of hyperglycemia in the db/db mice. *Phytother Res.*1992; 6:25-28.

20. Nyarko, A. K., Sittie, A. A., Addy, M.E. The basis for the anti-hyperglycemic activity of Indigofera arrecta. *Phytother Res.* 1993; 7:1-4

21. Nyarko, A. K., Ankrah, N. A., Ofosuhene, M., Sittie, A. A. Acute and subchronic evaluation of Indigofera arrecta: Absence of both toxicity

and modulation of selected cytochrome P450 isozymes in ddY mice. *Phytother Res.* 1999; 13: 686-688.

22. Nyarko, A. K., Asare-Anane, H., Ofosuhene, M., Addy, M. E. Extract of Ocimum canum lowers blood glucose and facilitates insulin release by isolated pancreatic -islet cells. *Phytomedicine.* 2002; 9: 346-351.

23. Okine, L. K. N., Nyarko, A. K., Osei-Kwabena, N., Barnes, F., Ofosuhene, M. The anti-diabetic activity of the herbal preparation ADD-199 in mice: A comparative study with two oral hypoglycaemic drugs. *J Ethnopharmacol.* 2005; 97: 31-38.

24. Drazen, J. M. Pharmacology of leukotriene receptor antagonists and 5-lipoxygenase inhibitors in the management of asthma. *Pharmacotherapy.*1997; 17: S22-S30.

25. Dogne, J. M., de Leval, X., Benoit, P., Rolin, S., Pirotte, B., Masereel, B. Therapeutic potential of thromboxane inhibitors in asthma. *Expert Opin Investigational Drugs.* 2002; 11: 275-81.

26. Coffey, M., Peters-Golden, M. Extending the understanding of leukotrienes in asthma. Curr Opin Allergy Clin Immunol. 2003; 3: 57-63.

27. Addy, M. E., Nyarko, A. K. Anti-anaphylactic properties of Thonningia sanguinea. *Planta Medica.* 1985; 51: 361-365.

28. Coffin, J. M. HIV population dynamics in vivo: implications for the genetic variations, pathogenesis and therapy. *Science.* 1995; 267: 483–488.

29. Cherry, C. L., Wesselingh, S.L. Nucleoside analogues and HIV: the combined cost to mitochondria. *J Antimicrob Chemother.* 2003; 51: 1091-1093.

30. Coffin, J. M. Retroviridae and their replication. In: Fields, B.N, Knipes, D.M, et al. eds.*Virology,* second ed. 1990. New York: Raven Press. p.1437–1499.

31. Erickson, J., Neidhart, D. .,VanDrie, J. *et al.* Design, activity and 2.8 A crystal structure of a C2 symmetric inhibitor complex to HIV-1protease. *Science.* 1990; 249: 527–533.

32. Kempf, D. J., Marsh, K. C., Paul, D. A. *et al.* Antiviral and pharmacokinetic properties of C2 symmetric inhibitors of the human immunodeficiency virus type1 protease. *Antimicrob Agents Chemother.*1991; 35: 2209–2214.

33. Lech, W. J., Wang, G., Yang, Y. L. *et al.* In vivo sequence diversity of the protease of human immuno-deficiency virus type1:presence of protease inhibitor-resistant variants in untreated subjects. *J Virol.* 1996;70: 2038–2043.

34. Delgoda, R., Westlake, A. C. G. Herbal interactions involving cytochrome P450 enzymes. *Toxicol Rev.* 2004; 23: 239-249.

35. Zafar, A., Sharif, M. D. Pharmacokinetics, metabolism, and metabolism of atypical antipsy-chotics in special populations. Primary care companion *J Clin Psychiatry.* 2003; 5: 22-25.

36. Pea, F., Furlanut, M. Pharmacokinetic aspects of treating infections in the intensive care unit: focus on drug interactions. *Clin Pharmacokinet.* 2001; 40: 833-868.

37. Lahoz, A., Donato, M. T., Montero, S., Castell, J. V., Gomez-Lechon, M. J. A new in vitro approach for the simultaneous determination of phase I and phase II enzymatic activities of human hepatocyte preparations. *Rapid Commun Mass Spectrom.* 2008; 22: 240-244.

# Chapter 22
# Lessons on Provider and Community Perceptions of Why Women Do Not Use Free Delivery Services in Ghana

*Daniel Kojo Arhinful, Sawudatu Zakariah, Akoto Margaret, Armar-Klemesu, Barbara Mallet and Banyana Madi*

## Introduction

Majority of women across Africa remain without access to maternal care. The variety of obstacles to improved maternal health includes cost and other access issues that prevent women from using the available resources.[1] To overcome the problem, governments in Africa continue to explore and implement various strategies to finance maternal health. Concerns that user fees reduce access to services among the poor, particularly in resource-constrained countries, have led to the promotion of fee-exemption mechanisms in order to protect those unable to pay for services. Most governments and partners therefore introduce exemptions and waivers to ensure that particular groups of the population have access to appropriate health care.[2] Available evidence, however, suggests that exemptions may not effectively ensure access among the poor because most exemption mechanisms are weakly defined and poorly implemented.[3,4,5]

The safe motherhood movement has, since the 1980s, taken the reduction of maternal mortality as its top priority. While there are some concerns that safe motherhood often comes as merely a subset of other programmes like child survival or reproductive health,[6] there is consensus about its importance. Skilled care at delivery is one of the strategies identified as key contributors to the reduction of maternal mortality.[7,8,9]

Ensuring skilled care for all births is a prerequisite for making sure that women who develop complications get timely emergency obstetric care. However, available evidence indicates that in sub-Saharan Africa, a region that accounts for nearly half of the 529,000 maternal deaths each year, there is an acute shortage of skilled attendants. According to population-based surveys, the percentage of deliveries with skilled attendants in the region between 1990 and 2000 only increased from 40% to 43%.[10]

Studies have noted that many factors complicate women's access to skilled care in sub-Saharan Africa. Poor women in particular tend to be excluded from health care by barriers that are difficult to overcome.[11] Women often give birth at home because of the prohibitive cost of medical care or cultural beliefs that promote home-based delivery. Difficult geographic terrain and limited transportation may present obstacles to reaching a skilled attendant. Apart from the lack of skilled providers, some people also lack confidence in the health system. The situation is aggravated by resource-constrained health systems that offer few incentives for skilled providers to remain in their country of origin, particularly in rural areas.[10] Furthermore, cultural and educational barriers that prevent poor women from revealing their pregnancy status and using maternal care services exacerbates the problem.[11]

It has also been noted that health workers' behaviour towards their clients play a role in women's use of skilled care.[12] Several studies have indicated that problems related to provider behaviour and attitudes in maternity care constitute major barriers to utilization of skilled care at childbirth in both developed and developing countries that affect access, compliance, quality and effectiveness of maternity care.[13,14,15,16] The examples include neglect, verbal abuse, and intentional humiliation of women during childbirth in many countries.

The government of Ghana introduced a fee exemption policy on deliveries in September 2003 in the four most deprived regions of the country, namely, the Central, Northern, Upper East and Upper West regions. In April 2005, it was extended to the remaining six regions of the country. The aim of the policy was to reduce financial barriers to using maternity services. The expected output was that the policy will lead to a greater number of supervised deliveries, and thereby, a reduction in maternal mortality rates. The policy was introduced in line with the Ghana Poverty Reduction Strategy (GPRS) and the health sector's 5-year-programme-of-work (5YPOW) which aimed to bridge inequalities in health among the regions. Funding was provided through the Highly Indebted Poor Countries (HIPC) debt relief that Ghana benefited from during the period. Payment for services for this initial policy was effected through the local government administration and later through the Ministry of Health.

In 2005, the Initiative for Maternal Mortality Programme Assessment (Immpact) Ghana evaluated the delivery policy, focusing on the process of implementation; how the policy had affected utilization, quality of services and health and non-health outcomes for households.[3] As part of the evaluation, a qualitative study was conducted to examine service provider and community perceptions of the policy in relation to quality of maternal services and barriers to seeking delivery care at the health facility.

In order to overcome implementation difficulties the government in 2008 decided to consolidate the free maternity policy for women by integrating it into the National Health Insurance Scheme (NHIS). Making the free maternal services part of the NHIS was expected "to ensure consistency in strategies for financing clinical care, and to support the longer-term objective of achieving 100% coverage of Ghanaians under the NHIS". In particular, the view of government was that the arrangement was expected "to systematically register all pregnant women to enable them to take advantage of 'free' antenatal, delivery and post-natal services at the time that they require them". Simultaneously, health facilities would be guaranteed reimbursement for services provided.

This paper presents findings on women's attitude and use of skilled care in the context of the initial free delivery policy funded under HIPC, in order to provide demand-side lessons that are still relevant for the attainment of the objective of enrolling all pregnant women to enable them receive "free" antenatal, delivery and post-natal services. The specific objective was to examine providers' and women's perceptions of the free delivery policy and their views about factors affecting utilization of skilled care in the context of the free delivery policy.

# Approach

## Study location and context

The evaluation of the free delivery policy by Immpact was conducted in the Central and Volta regions from October 2005 to April 2006. The Central Region was chosen to reflect the experiences of the four economically poorest regions where the delivery exemption scheme was started while the Volta Region was chosen to reflect the experiences of the remaining six regions that joined the scheme later. Findings reported in this paper are from two districts, one each in the Central and Volta regions of Ghana. These two districts were purposively selected, matched for poverty rates and other characteristics. Three communities were selected from each district as follows: the district capital where the district hospital is located; a community distant from the district capital that had a health centre; and a rural community without a health facility.

In the Central Region, Agona District, with Agona Swedru as its capital, was selected. Agona District has an estimated population of about 158,955 people, (2000 Census) with a growth rate of 2.1%. The main economic activities are fishing and farming. The district has a total of 31 health facilities of which 22 are administered by the Ghana Health Service (GHS); two are mission and four are private facilities. The health facilities are not evenly distributed across the district and therefore, monthly outreach services are encouraged in all the remote areas.

The Kpando District was chosen in the Volta Region. The district has an estimated population of 121,794 (2000 census) spread across 205 communities, with a growth rate of 2.1%. The main economic activities are fishing and some amount of farming at the subsistence level. Trading, pottery, woodcarving and making of firearms are other activities. The district capital is Kpando.

## Ethical approval and participant consent

The Scientific and Technical Committee and the Institutional Review Board of the Noguchi Memorial Institute for Medical Research, University of Ghana, granted approval for this study. The Regional and District Health Directorates of the two study regions also gave their consent for the study to be carried out in their respective districts. Written and verbal consent was also received from each of the health institutions and study subjects and the anonymity and confidentiality of their participation was assured.

## Participants and data collection techniques

Sample selection was conceived to capture participants who were informed and/or aware of the free delivery policy to provide useful insights on the perceived barriers to the provision and use of delivery services by women. Selection of study participants was, therefore, mainly purposive. For the provider aspect of the study, 19 in-depth interviews were conducted with purposively selected key informants in the two districts. The informants comprised 4 medical officers, 13 midwives, one nurse/midwife and one ward assistant. Two of the medical officers were district health managers while the remaining two were heads of the district hospitals studied. Provider interviews were conducted mainly in English and tape recorded. Notes were also taken to augment the transcripts. In addition to the in-depth interviews, a group discussion was held with five midwives in one district hospital. Providers were recruited at their places of work. Written consent to participate in the study was obtained from all those who participated. The interview and discussion topics covered providers' perceptions of the free delivery policy; views about factors affecting utilization of skilled care in the context of the free delivery policy; views about the standard of care provided in the context of free delivery care in Ghana; and views on factors affecting motivation to provide good quality care under the free delivery policy.

Recruitment of community members (users, non-users and local opinion leaders) took place in the community using key informants initially and then by snowballing methods. A fair representation of socio economic and demographic backgrounds, including urban and rural, was covered. Most of the mothers had attended antenatal care at least once during pregnancy and some had experience with both home trained birth attendants (TBA) and formal facility deliveries. The in-depth interview and focus group guides were structured along major themes with topics covering issues of awareness, impressions and problems of the free delivery policy; quality of care; barriers to seeking skilled care; views about the TBA and hospital delivery.

Before the main study, a pilot was conducted in Kasoa in the Effutu District in the Central Region and Tsito in the Ho District in the Volta Region. The actual data collection was preceded by community orientation sessions to enable the field team members to familiarize themselves with the communities, and create awareness of their activities. The sessions also aimed to gain acceptance from the elders and people in the community and to establish key contacts with persons who helped to facilitate the work of the team during the actual data collection. Activities included courtesy calls on the local authorities and other community stakeholders as well as health workers, review of maternity records at health facilities and generally observing and learning about the cultural life of the people. Data collection was between November 2005 and April 2006.

## Data analysis

Data analysis was done using both electronic and manual procedures. It started with transcription of tapes, which began concurrently with data collection. For quality control purposes, transcripts were read and checked against the original recording. The field team also held a debriefing meeting at the end of each day's field sessions to discuss and review performance and the information obtained. Data were subsequently managed with the aid of NVIVO[17] software for qualitative analysis.

# Results

## Socio-demographic characteristics of women FGD participants

A total of 11 focus group discussions, comprising five in the Central Region and six in the Volta Region were conducted with an average of 10 participants per group discussion. In all, about 163 mothers with ages ranging between 15 and 46 years participated in the study. They included both users of TBA services and users of health facility delivery services. Most (90.6%) of them were married and parity was from one to 10 children with a mean of three children. The ages of the last child ranged from one month to five years. The majority (57.8%) of the mothers had basic education up to the junior secondary school level while 17.2% studied up to senior secondary school, technical or vocational level. Another 17.2% had no formal education at all and the remaining 7.8% had primary education. The majority (63.7%) of respondents were engaged in farming and trading while about 18.2% earned a living as seamstresses and hairdressers. About 14.3% were unemployed and the remaining 3.9% were clerical staff.

## Perceptions of the free delivery policy and its implementation

The overwhelming view of providers and mothers was that the free delivery policy was good and acceptable because it removed the financial barrier to skilled care for women who previously could not afford the cost of delivery and thereby encouraged them to deliver at health facilities. Most mothers, especially in poor rural communities, described it as a very welcome financial relief. A key outcome of the policy stressed by mothers and providers alike was that it made it possible for some women, particularly the rural poor, to access timely delivery care. Timely reporting, according to providers, also reduced the number of women arriving at facilities with complications and potentially decreased maternal and infant deaths when the policy was fully operational. The cumulative effect of the policy, according to providers, was that it resulted in increased hospital utilization. Some were of the opinion that increased attendance at health facilities was partly because of a drift of some women from TBA services. The policy was also credited with an important psychological benefit in the form of health facilities being spared the embarrassment of hitherto detaining women who were unable to afford the cost of delivery services.

> *The policy was fine because when they come, we don't have any stress. We just pick the things we use on the patient. The patient gets well and just goes away, but when the patient is sick and the patient cannot afford, it gives us headache... stress! You go to your work site and all the things are there and you just pick them and work because you are here to save lives. ...* Midwife, Volta Region

However, the foregoing positive views about the policy were not without concerns. The most commonly expressed concern of most providers was the erratic inflow of funds to sustain the policy. The policy was implemented through a mechanism of reimbursement based on receipts submitted. Reimbursements were, however, inadequate and/or unduly delayed. Bills submitted took three months or more to be processed and honoured. That made it difficult for facilities to implement the policy because by the time money was received the outstanding expesnses, could not be completely defrayed.

## Views about factors affecting utilization of skilled care by women

Myriad and interesting views were expressed by providers and mothers to explain the attitudes of women and their acceptance of use of skilled care under the free delivery policy. In the first place, even though the cost of care at the point of delivery was taken care of by the exemption policy, women had to incur other expenses related to delivery. This was seen as a major barrier to seeking facility delivery. These other expenses include the cost of specific items women were required to take along to the health facility during delivery such as baby clothes, cot sheets, cost of transport to the facility and facility-related costs such as laboratory investigations and drugs. Both providers and women identified these additional costs to be posing problems to women. However, some providers were of the view that women who complain of such items because of poverty are usually those who have uncontrolled and unregulated pregnancies and births.

Another barrier to women, frequently mentioned by both providers and women, was the difficult rural terrain and long distances to health facilities and the associated problems of securing means of transport to facilities. A facility non-user in the Volta Region depicted it during an in-depth interview as follows:

> What I want to say is that transportation is a problem for us here. You will go through hell before getting vehicle to go to the hospital. I am always scared of travelling on the river by boat so the 4 times I attended antenatal, I had to go round with vehicles. I will appreciate it if you could solve the transportation problem here or put up a facility here for us.

Reasons associated with health services systemic factors, particularly limited equipment and infrastructure, were also cited. Providers made reference to limited space and facilities at the labour ward. One midwife at a health centre in the Volta Region lamented this situation as follows:

> We are not ok with the delivery facilities because all these things were brought here during the colonial time; you will notice that they are very old, even our mattresses, you can see that they are not good... Besides the delivery wards, we do not get the delivery kits as expected.

Findings on perceived value of skilled care of women and how it influenced their care-seeking behaviour were varied and revealing. On one hand, the perception of users about facility delivery was that it is a place for expert care where one is given the required drugs to control pain and excessive bleeding and where unforeseen complications and emergencies can be managed. Other facility users were simply confident about facility delivery services because their parents and other relatives had had their deliveries in health facilities with no problems.

On the other hand, the views of users of traditional birth attendants (TBA) about skilled care was that health facilities are meant for only mothers with pregnancy or delivery complications. In their opinion, therefore, one need not go to a facility for delivery unless one had a problem with a pregnancy or labour. To them, some mothers experience a lot of difficulty during labour and need the intervention of medical experts. In addition, this group of mothers was of the view that facility delivery was meant for a certain group of women such as women pregnant with their first child, women pregnant with twins and mothers with more than four children. They also believed that one only needed the services of the facility if there were no TBAs in the community or when a TBA had difficulty in delivering and referred the case.

Poor staff attitude on one hand and confidence of some women in traditional birth attendants were also mentioned by both providers and mothers as factors that make some potential clients in the community less motivated to patronise skilled care services at the facility. Accounts of facility users indicated that midwives sometimes shout at them to push when they are struggling in labour. Some mothers, predomi-nantly TBA users, indicated that providers were sometimes rude to them and explained that some people by nature are not caring and if one is unfortunate to meet such persons during labour then one is likely to receive bad treatment from them. In one district, for example, it was revealed that some mothers opted to travel to distant facilities to deliver their babies in order to avoid bad treatment from staff in facilities closer to them. Some women, however, attributed negative attitudes of providers to difficult and uncooperative clients who do not follow the instructions of the providers. In corroborating the view of poor staff attitude, a doctor who was a district director in the Central Region, briefly explained the situation thus:

> I think we need to learn to provide client care. We just provide service but we don't take time to understand the client before providing service. Sometimes in the midst of pain, you are asking the poor woman to push; this brings us to the issue of staff attitude.

In contrast to poor staff attitudes, a number of reasons were given to explain the favourable disposition towards TBAs which serves as a pull factor. According to some mothers interviewed, the charges of

TBA services were much lower than the additional charges one had to incur in the health facility under the free delivery policy. Furthermore, the TBA charges were considered flexible so one can use a lifetime to settle the debt. These aside, mothers do not need to buy items such as cot sheets baby clothes when they deliver with the TBA. An interesting finding was that trained TBAs were perceived by some mothers as being representatives of midwives, and conceived as able and fully competent to handle all deliveries. As such, mothers who lived in communities where there are health facilities felt very confident patronizing the services of trained TBAs.

Free delivery was intended to shift births to facilities for skilled care and this appeared to have been the case. Containing the additional workload from increased attendance at various levels was described as a tedious and difficult task and sometimes compromising. Nonetheless, most providers held the view that quality of care was not affected because drugs and supplies were available. Several providers explained that despite the increased pressure, they were able to maintain the level of quality in service delivery through the efficient use of existing overstretched resources. However, non-users of skilled care did not agree with this assertion but rather indicated that they distrusted and/or lacked confidence in the quality of care in general and feared the worst under the free delivery policy.

> I won't go because when you go to the hospital to deliver you are not given sufficient or good care and as it is even free of charge, I believe the quality of care will be worse; because they know they can't take money from you, they do just what pleases them so you will not get the kind of care you will get at home. I will never say that because it is free I will get up and go to deliver at the hospital. No I won't; I am pleased with TBA delivery (Non user, C/R).

From a cultural standpoint, a number of problems were also identified. One of these was related to negative attitudes and social misconceptions. For example, it was explained that some women attend a health facility only if their husbands or mothers-in-law agree. Besides, it is still believed in some communities that women who have difficulty in labour are those unfaithful to their husbands.

In summary, the general view of informants was that although free delivery led to improved access for women, persistent obstacles such as transport and other service costs, geographic access, poor staff attitude, cultural and social barriers and preference for traditional birth attendants remain.

## Discussion

This study provides qualitative insights of providers and women into the effects of the free delivery policy on the provision and utilization of skilled care at delivery in the Central and Volta Regions with implications for the entire country. The use of mixed qualitative methods involving in-depth interviews and focus group discussions in the study was intended to maximize the advantages of the two methods. Multiple methods helped in checking the accuracy of information, as individual interviews were sometimes used to identify pertinent issues, which were then followed up in the group situation or vice versa. The qualitative approach enabled study informants to freely raise issues related to the policy and skilled care that were relevant to them. The similarity in the views of providers interviewed however, did not make it conducive to structure the analysis more systematically by type of provider.

The findings indicate that the policy of fee exemption was found to be beneficial because it led to timely access to care for women, particularly the poor, who otherwise could not have afforded care. When the policy was operational, it not only encouraged women to deliver at health facilities but also made it easier and/or convenient for providers to deliver maternal health care services to those who needed them and made it to facilities since the payment for care was already secured. Evidence of the favourable reaction of some mothers leading to the timely reporting and increased facility utilization when the policy was fully operational suggests that cost is an important consideration in decision making by mothers or families as to whether or not to use skilled care although it is not the only one. The findings here indicate that the free delivery policy was perceived to have led to increased supervised deliveries, thereby achieving one of its expected outcomes.

Findings indicate that not all mothers took advantage of the free delivery policy. Mothers' views on facility delivery greatly influenced their decisions to either seek skilled care at delivery or not. Where mothers perceived the facility as a place where only complications and emergency care are sought, then they would naturally not seek facility care until they experience an emergency situation at labour. This perception is a major setback to seeking skilled care and has serious risk implications for the health of prospective mothers and therefore needs to be tackled appropriately. The finding also shows the importance of social attitudes in family decision making to use skilled care.

It could be inferred from the findings that from a social perspective, the context of the fee exemption policy improved community perceptions regarding the advantages of facility delivery or skilled care for women in labour. The evidence thus suggests the fee exemption policy considerably enhanced family decision making to seek skilled care and thereby weakened some of the biases and social influences that contribute to the first delay.[18]

The findings also indicate that the policy did not change non-users negative perceptions about the attitudes of health workers. In one district for example, facility users opted to deliver in an adjoining district hospital as a result of dissatisfaction with staff attitudes. A previous study in southern Ghana reported that 44% of Ghanaian women delivered by health professionals explained that three major problems with the maternal care were lack of staff, poor attitudes among health workers and lack of community preparedness.[10] Another study on midwives' attitudes towards women in labour also reported that although women expected kind, courteous and professional treatment, health workers shouted, were rude and refused to offer assistance and in some cases threatened women in labour.[12] In order to tackle the problem of negative staff attitudes, this study identifies with the recommendation that health staff should receive training to improve their interpersonal skills in counselling women, learning to communicate well and showing sensitivity to different cultures. It is important to also add that the context within which the free delivery policy took place as reported here was characterized by increased workload in resource-constrained facilities. There was also undue stress on staff without commensurate increase in expected motivation. In the light of the findings here, it is essential that the attitudinal problems of health workers be addressed in tandem with the difficult conditions in which they work.

Even though some mothers reacted favourably towards the policy, as evidenced by increased facility utilization, the findings of this study strongly indicate that persistent obstacles to women exist in the form of geographic access and transport to facilities. Social and cultural beliefs also continue to impede the use of services. Afful has noted that among other factors, poverty, unavailability of transport, costs of health care as well as socio-cultural beliefs were barriers in northern Ghana.[19] The importance of the influence of socio demographic and cultural barriers are underscored by the fact that an estimated 56% of Ghanaians live in rural areas[20] where health facilities and other social services are limited or non-existent. What that translates into is that in terms of access, a good majority of the poor still remain far removed from benefiting from the free delivery policy.

One of the major setbacks to the policy that characterized its implementation, as reported by some providers, was the irregular release of funds and the inability of the government to reimburse them regularly for services provided. One school of thought among providers was that targeting women in most need and unable to pay for services in the design of the scheme would have allowed a prudent use of the limited financial resources. It is noteworthy that the irregularity of funds that characterised the policy also led to some suggestions for the integration of the delivery scheme in the National Health Insurance Scheme to provide a more sustainable source of funding.

It is important to note also that the free delivery policy was introduced partly in response to poverty as a major contributory factor to inequalities in maternal health care service utilization. Yet the policy did not factor targeting of poor women into the implementation. Other findings of the evaluation of the free delivery policy published elsewhere concluded that all women benefited equally from the exemption policy irrespective of status.[21] The lesson there aligns with the view that policy efforts that cast maternal health in the context of poverty alleviation and the reduction of inequalities require recognition that inequalities exist.[3] In summary, findings in this paper confirm other observations that exemptions alone may not effectively ensure access among the poor because informal fees and other costs associated with seeking and receiving services are not alleviated by such mechanisms.[2]

## Conclusions

The foregoing discussion provides a number of policy lessons for delivery care in Ghana:

- The cost of services is clearly not the full story about women's motivation to use skilled care. Geographical and cultural barriers are still crucial. Special efforts to focus on indirect barriers such as difficult geographic terrain, transport costs and cultural factors also need priority attention.
- Women's care-seeking behaviour in some cases was unlikely to change under free delivery because of negative experiences, perceptions and/or misconceptions about facility delivery care. It is, therefore, of prime importance to enhance efforts aimed at getting midwives and other health care providers, particularly, in the public health system to change negative attitudes in order to encourage pregnant women to use facility care if skilled care for all is to become a reality.
- The free delivery policy resulted in additional workload and increased pressure on facilities. Mechanisms should have been put in place to ensure that undue pressure was not put on staff in order to ensure that quality was not compromised.
- The system for managing the implementation of the policy was affected by lack of and/or concrete planning and coordination of the various implementing bodies. A key lesson from this review, therefore, is that not only are prudent planning and management essential for the success of official policies conceived at the highest political level but also the commitment and accountability of staff at the frontline service delivery level are crucial for its success.

# Acknowledgements

This work was undertaken as part of an international research programme—IMMPACT (Initiative for Maternal Mortality Programme Assessment) – funded by the Bill & Melinda Gates Foundation, the UK Department for International Development, the European Commission and USAID. The funders have no responsibility for the information provided or views expressed in this paper. The views expressed herein are solely those of the authors.

We would like to acknowledge the assistance of all members of the research team at the Noguchi Memorial Institute for Medical Research, Ghana, and the University of Aberdeen, Scotland. Our appreciation goes to Prof. David Ofori-Adjei for his comments on earlier drafts of the paper. We also wish to express our gratitude to staff and communities in the study areas who gave time to share their expertise and knowledge with us.

# References

1. World Health Organisation. Maternal Health: Investing in the Lifeline of Healthy Societies and Economies. Africa Progress Panel Policy Brief; September 2010. Available at: http://www.who.int/pmnch/topics/maternal/app_maternal_health_english.pdf. Accessed on 21 August 2013.

2. Kivumbi, G. W, Kintu, F. (2002) Exemptions and waivers from cost sharing: ineffective safety nets in decentralized districts in Uganda. *Health Policy and Planning* 17 (Suppl. 1): 64–71.

3. Sharma, S., Smith, S., Sonneveldt, S., Pine, M., Dayaratna, V., Sanders, R. (2005) Formal and Informal Fees for Maternal Health Care Services in Five Countries: Policies, Practices, and Perspectives. USAID Policy Working Paper Series No. 16; June 2005.

4. Schneider, P. and Dmytraczenko, T. Insights for Implementers: Improving Access to Maternal Health Care through Insurance. 2003. Partners for Health Reformplus Brief No. 3. Washington DC: USAID.

5. Bitrán, R., Giedion, U. (2003). Waivers and Exemptions for Health Services in Developing Countries, Social Protection. Discussion Paper Series, No.0308; 2003. Washington DC: The World Bank.

6. AbouZahr, C. (2003) Safe Motherhood: a brief history of the global movement 1947-2002. *British Medical Bulletin.* 2003. 67: 13-25.

7. WHO. The role of the health services in preventing maternal deaths. In: Royston, E. and Armstrong, S. eds. Preventing Maternal Deaths. 1989. Geneva: WHO, 153-183.

8. Family Care International (2002) Skilled Care during Childbirth: Policy Brief.

9. de Bernis, L., Sherratt, D. R., AbouZahr, C., van Lerberghe, W. (2003) Skilled attendants for pregnancy, childbirth and postnatal care. British Medical Bulletin 67: 39-57

10. UNFPA. Into good hands: Progress reports from the field. 2004. New York: UNFPA.

11. D'Ambruoso, L., Abbey, M., Hussein, J. Please, understand when I cry out in pain: women's accounts of maternity services during labour and delivery in Ghana. *BMC Public Health* 2005 5: 140.

12. Moore, M., Armbruster, D., Graeff, J., Copeland, R. Assessing the "caring" behaviours of skilled maternity care providers during labour and delivery: Experience from Kenya and Bangladesh. 2002. Washington DC: 2002. Washington DC: The CHANGE Project; The Academy for Educational Development/The Manoff Group.

13. Di Olivera, A., Diniz, S. and Schraiber, L. (2002) Violence against women in a health care setting. *The Lancet.* 359: 1681-1685.

14. Andaleeb, S.S. Service quality perceptions and patient satisfaction: A study of hospitals in a developing country. Social Science and Medicine 2001.52: 1359-1370.

15. Andaleeb, S.S. Public and private hospitals in Bangladesh: service quality and predictors of hospital choice. Health policy and Planning. 2000. 15 (1): 95–102.

16. NVivo, © QSR International Pty Ltd 2013 http://www.qsrinternational.com/default.aspx.

17. Thaddeus, S., Maine, D. Too far to walk: maternal mortality in context. *Social Science and Medicine* 1994. 38:1091-1110.

18. Afful, T. M. (2004) Safe deliveries in Kassena-Nankana District in Northern Ghana: A study to determine factors influencing the use of health facilities for deliveries by pregnant women. (Unpublished MA thesis, University of Copenhagen, Denmark).

19. Ghana Statistical Service. 2000 Population and Housing Census: Summary Report of Final Results. 2002. Accra: GSS.

20. Asante, F. A., Chikwama, C., Daniels, A. Evaluating the economic outcomes of the policy of fee exemption for maternal delivery care in Ghana; *Ghana Medical Journal* 2007. 41(3): 110–117.

# Index

## A

Acid-fast bacilli (AFB) 112,119,

Acquired immunodeficiency syndrome (AIDS) xxxiv, xxxviii, 115, 151, 155, 156, 218, 220-224, 228, 229, 260, 276, 282, 284

Acute flaccid paralysis (AFP) xxiii, 208, 210, 231, 232, 235-239, 242

Ada-Foah xxv, 206-208, 212-215, 217-219

Africa 5, 7, 11, 16, 17, 19-21, 27, 30-34, 37, 43, 44, 48-50, 65, 66, 75, 77, 91-95, 103

Alchornea cordifolia 96, 99, 101-104

Allelic 59, 64, 66, 68-71, 73, 74

Amodiaquine 17, 20, 22, 23, 34, 103

Amoeba 131-135, 137

Anaemia 11, 26, 30, 33, 34, 37, 42, 44, 48, 55, 100

Anaphylaxis 282

Anopheles 81, 83, 87, 90, 92, 190, 191, 195, 197, 202-204; Funestus v, 78, 82-85, 92, 93; Gambiae v, 78, 81-85, 88, 92-94

Anophelines 81, 84

Antenatal care 295

Anti-asthmatic 277, 282

Antibodies 40, 42, 45, 46, 57, 59, 60, 61, 63, 64, 66, 76

Anti-diabetes 276, 277

Antigens x, xvii, xx, 16, 39, 41, 45, 46, 57-66, 75, 76, 81

Anti-HIV 222, 277, 282, 285

Anti-inflammatory 174

Antimalarial iv, xiv, xvii, 7-17, 32, 38, 68, 77, 95-105

Antiplasmodial 96, 97, 100, 102-104

Antiretroviral therapy (ART) 220, 222, 224-229 Anti-TB drug 112

Artemether 17

Artesunate 17, 20, 22, 23, 33, 48, 101

Ascaris lumbricoides 173, 183, 187, 206

## B

BED HIV-1 222

Bednet 48, 91

Biofilms 137

Biting 82-84, 87, 90

Buruli ulcer xxi, xxiii, xxiv, xxxiv, 131, 132, 138-141, 148, 149, 153, 155, 156-160, 163, 170-172; BU lesion 155; BU-related morbidity 168; classification of BU stages : Nodule 142, 143, 150, 159; Oedema 143, 150, 152, 188, 252; Papule 142, 150, 159; Plaque 142, 143;

## C

Candidates x, xvi, 57, 58, 98, 100

Carbanotes 82

Cells xiii, xiv, 23, 36, 38-40, 47-49, 51-54, 56, 58, 96, 99, 100

Chemoprevention 21, 27, 33

Chemotherapy x, 15, 19, 78

Chikungunya (virus) 256, 258

Chloroquine 8, 11, 13, 16, 17, 19, 20, 44, 66, 95, 96, 99-103

Chondroitin 38-40, 44-46

Circulating recombinant forms (CRFs) 220

Circumsporozoite 67, 76, 81

Clinical v, x, xiv-xvi, 4, 5, 8-10, 20, 21, 23, 26, 32-35, 38, 39, 48, 54, 55, 57, 59-64, 66, 67, 73, 75-78, 91, 98, 99, 102

Clonal v, 42, 63, 66, 67-71, 73

Co-infection xxxi, 155, 156, 173, 174, 177, 179, 182, 183, 187,188, 254

Colorimetric 97, 99, 101

Community-based volunteers 161, 162, 165, 169,

Contraindication 9

Control vi, ix, x, xii, xiii, xv, xvii, 4, 5, 7, 14, 15, 19-21, 23, 30, 32-34, 43,